DR. EICHENLAUB'S
HOME TONICS AND REFRESHERS
FOR DAILY *HEALTH* AND *VIGOR*

DR. EICHENLAUB'S
HOME TONICS
FOR DAILY *HEALTH*

PRENTICE-HALL, INC.

AND REFRESHERS
AND *VIGOR*

JOHN E. EICHENLAUB
M.D.

Englewood Cliffs, New Jersey

Second Printing, July 1963

PRINTED IN THE UNITED STATES OF AMERICA
21895—B&P

Every man who knows how to read has it in his power to magnify himself, to multiply the ways in which he exists, to make his life full, significant, and interesting.
—ALDOUS HUXLEY

Contents

1. Depend on natural food, not pills and potions
94, 2. Count food groups, not fuel values 95,
3. County 4-5-5 for greater vigor 96, 4. Eat often
for energy 99, 5. Use your quick-energy snacks to
fill your food count 99, 6. Boost reserve-energy
foods 100, 7. Replace table spreads, shortening and
fats or oils with quicker energy foods whenever possible 101, 8. Dodge chemically treated fats for long-
term tonic action 102, 9. Eat foods in a form you can
readily chew 103, 10. Regulate your bowels the
natural way 103, Summary 105.

Drugless stimulating drinks 110, Digestive tonics
112, Summary 115.

Nose 118, Ears 122, The mouth 124, The female
organs 126, Bowel 130, Summary 132.

Self-training 136, Equipment for better bone-balance
141, Exercises 149, Summary 152.

Air in cold weather 157, Comes the spring 162,
Air in warm weather 163, Breathed-in refreshers
165, Summary 166.

Light versus contrast 171, Other eye easers 176,
Summary 179.

Why "Natural" Tonics and Refreshers?

As a doctor, I've learned to respect drug firm chemists. When you sit at a child's bedside and watch death's forces rapidly retreat from a near-victory, you can't help applauding whatever turned the tide. But medical research and pharmacy spend their main effort combatting disease and injury, not improving zest and vigor. Few of their findings apply to daily life, and risks or side-effects quite tolerable during a fight for survival have no place among the well.

On the other hand, people without access to prescription drugs have sought ways of feeling better since the beginning of time. The safe, successful methods pass on through the generations, while the ineffective or risky ones die with disuse. The distillation of the ages has built a rich store of ways to build zest, to increase vigor, to restore energy after a tough day—methods you can use

11

in your own home, with little expenditure of time or money, whenever you want to feel your absolute best. That's why most of the tonics and refreshers in this book are "natural" instead of "manufactured."

There's a tremendous difference between feeling "all right" and feeling "really great." Even when no special miseries plague you, you can almost certainly *feel* better, *last out each day* better, and *tone up mental and physical abilities* you hardly know exist with the tonics and refreshers in this book. For instance, there's the state of mind and body so spectacular that experts call it *"the* tonic response"—a perked-up feeling which follows exercise, massage, hot baths and cold applications when suited exactly to your own body's needs. Unless you have actually experienced it, the words sound as exaggerated as descriptions of bright colors must seem to a blind man. Yet millions of devotees pursue this sensation each day, and almost anyone can discover it through the methods detailed in this book.

Yes, the sure-fire tonics listed in this book can help you feel really great. Of course, some of them work quickly, and others require a little time. The food program described in Chapter Six won't make you feel better the first day you try it, for instance, but inside three weeks you'll probably find yourself less tired by the end of the day, less liable to colds and other illnesses, and more efficient in everything you do. All without spending a dime on vitamin pills or supplements—natural foods from your usual grocery do the trick. Improved body poise and balance work in much the same way: no spectacular, overnight change, but a gradual improvement in vigor, endurance and physical attractiveness. Even exercise has a time-bomb effect. It adds to your vigor and improves your health over a period of weeks or months, in addition to giving immediate benefits.

No matter how well you tone yourself up, though, you'll sometimes find yourself tired, irritable, depressed or upset. A quick refresher can make a lot of difference. It can help you to finish a job when weariness has begun to get you down. It can perk you up for a pleasant evening at home or at a party when you feel fit for nothing more strenuous than a flop on the nearest couch or a few hours of boring TV. It can keep a smile on your face and a pleasant word on your lips when your husband, your wife, or your children would otherwise get on your nerves.

This book tells about several dozen refreshers, from perk-up baths to recreations which blow off emotional steam. A whole chapterful of refreshers depend solely on running water, ranging from a tub-shower routine to get you started in the morning *fast* to a tranquilizing, nerve-soothing bath that's just what every housewife needs after a rainy day with children underfoot. Chapter Two tells you how to revive, re-energize or tranquilize with rubdown techniques. It includes the Salt Glow, the Sponge Rub, and a variety of simplified, anyone-can-do-it forms of special massage. You'll find exercises to abolish leg-weariness in mere seconds when you get to Chapter Four, and in Chapter Seven ways to enjoy the lift of tea and coffee without sleepless nights or constipation. Relaxation techniques, breathing exercises, and simplified yoga have proved themselves through many centuries, while modern inventions like the electric light and the hand vibrator can also help perk you up. You can surround yourself with quick refreshers through Chapter Ten's suggestions on the air you breathe, Chapter Thirteen's hints on room decoration, and Chapter Fourteen's deskside or stay-at-home diversions.

These methods will make you feel more vigorous, more cheerful, more full of get-up-and-go. But if that isn't enough by itself, you'll find many measures specifically devoted to making you feel youthful. Cold sitz baths as a sexual tonic, special use of color to avoid brain-weariness and uplift your mood, rays and exercises to speed aging circulation—all these specific methods help to roll back many of old age's common manifestations and make you feel distinctly younger.

When you feel "great," the world is your oyster. You do better at any task from running machinery to amusing a sick child. You finish your day's work with something left over in the way of energy with which to enjoy activities of your own choice. You keep cheerful and hold your temper in check. Your body fights off diseases which might otherwise cause a good deal of discomfort, expense and lost time.

You may not reach that state overnight. But just the measures *you yourself* decide upon as pleasant, suitable additions to your daily life will almost certainly give you an immediate boost. If you apply the ideas that suit *you* among the many this book sets forth, you'll almost certainly feel better right away, and keep feeling better and better through the weeks to come.

Give these natural tonics a fair test. Start with those which cost no time or money—the routines that add perk-up effects to baths you would take for cleanliness anyway, the exercises you can do while riding a bus or waiting in your car for a stoplight to turn green. Move on to those that prove themselves with quick results—sheet baths, the salt glow, hot bouillon as an evening drink. Sample those which fulfill certain special needs—tension fighters, digestion aids, eyestrain easers and mood-lifting emotional outlets—which you can easily locate through this book's comprehensive index. By the time you install the time-bomb tonics in your daily routine, you'll know from vast experience that natural refreshers work—that almost every change you make in your daily life because of this book's advice will pay off in lasting energy, restored youthfulness, and enduring health.

CHAPTER ONE

Water Tonics
and Refreshers

You've heard men say that their favorite sport or outdoor exercise makes them feel "great." I used to wonder what they meant —sports and exercise were fun for me, but I just felt tired instead of rejuvenated afterward. Then the Park Board put up a locker room beside the nearby tennis courts. Instead of cooling off for half or three-quarters of an hour on the ride home before taking a bath, I went straight from a fast, hard game to the showers. Hot blood still raced through my skin after my bath, so I turned on the cold spray. After a gasp or so from the first shock, the water felt warm as fresh milk and the hard needle spray seemed like a gentle, soothing caress. And afterwards, I did feel "great!" My brain felt clearer, my step more springy and my mood one of simultaneous keen interest and tranquility.

What happened? Just the normal tonic effect—the effect that you can personally experience *today*—of a proper hot-cold application. Like myself, you may have missed experiencing this effect through the years, perhaps only because of a few minutes' delay between the steps required to achieve it, perhaps because you've omitted some simple preliminary aid.

YOU CAN TONE UP WITH SPECIAL BATHS

You can enjoy substantial tonic effects from simple water treatments right in your own home and at virtually no cost in either money or effort, either with or without exercise, massage and other aids. Hot and cold water, with enough pressure behind them to activate swirling or sprays, can stimulate your mind and body or soothe and relax them. Water treatments can invigorate

16

you, raise your spirits, and make you feel literally "great." You'll find the necessary techniques detailed in the next few pages.

Water treatments: emotions in reverse. When you become either upset or exhilarated, your skin's blood vessels, sweat glands and hair follicle muscles (which tighten to make gooseflesh) signal your emotional state the way your dog's tail signals his pleasure when you pet him. But there's one difference: you can't crank up a dog's spirits by waving his tail, while the nerves attached to your skin and its expressive organs carry impulses both ways. These impulses don't reproduce full-fledged emotion, but they generate considerable emotion-mimicking bodily and psychologic change. You enjoy the strength of fear or anger, the exhilaration of delight or the peaceful repose of contentment almost at will, without the unpleasant or enervating aspects which often accompany rampant emotion itself.

THE PERK-UP, PEP-UP TONIC RESPONSE

The most commonly sought tonic response brings out your body's defensive forces without the stress of actual assault, like a gala military parade with no risk of battle. You feel stronger, look healthier, and get a real lift in mood because your mind and body get the boost the Good Lord designed to help them through times of trouble without being first pushed down by adversity. And at no real cost to you—the resources you mobilize with tonic routines actually become stronger through use.

Before you can experience a real tonic response, you have to meet two conditions:

1. Your circulation to both skin and muscles must be vigorous. This means that your body must be thoroughly warm, and that either exercise or friction from massage or moving water must have stimulated your muscles.
2. Something must stimulate large areas of your body

in a way which stirs protective mechanisms without actually causing pain or harm.

Preliminaries are absolute *musts*. A cold shower or plunge by itself does nothing but chill you. Moreover, a few minutes in a cool room or breeze beforehand often ruins your responsiveness to cold by driving blood away from your skin surface. You need at least two hours of seventy-two degree or greater warmth before any ordinary hot-cold tonic routine will work. Even at seventy-two, you may need to wear thermal underwear or an extra sweater and drink a cup of hot cocoa to get thoroughly warm. Deliberate exercise or physical work also helps to stir your skin's circulation.

Tub-shower routine. A further warm-up in an ordinary tub makes your skin much more responsive. Prepare by putting a washcloth and a pint or so of cold water in a basin near your tub and by filling the tub with water at 94 degrees, measuring temperature with a good bath or candy thermometer. Add moderately hotter water (110-120 degrees) until the bath temperature reaches 105. Do not let the hot water flowing into the tub strike your skin for fear of burns. Soak in the tub at 105 degrees for about ten minutes. Keep your washcloth wet with cold water from the separate basin, and apply to your forehead or the back of your neck. This controls congestion, which might otherwise cause ringing in the ears or headache. End the hot bath promptly if you find yourself becoming giddy, feeling nauseated or suffering other adverse effects. Such difficulties occur very rarely, but should not be ignored.

After ten minutes in a hot tub, your skin should look pinkish. Your muscles and nerves should feel distinctly relaxed. Now let the tub drain out and take a short shower, starting with lukewarm water and regulating the temperature steadily toward the cold side. With each temperature shift, turn so that the shower stream hits every part of your body and rub yourself vigorously with the palms of both hands in the areas where the water strikes. You may gasp for a breath or two as the water gets really cold, but that phase will pass in a few seconds and your skin will feel quite warm again. When warmth and healthy pinkness reach their maximum, or when you begin to feel cold and your skin forms gooseflesh, turn off the shower and rub yourself briskly with a warm dry towel. After your body is reasonably dry, switch to another towel and rub briskly again from head to toe, then put on a warm robe or clothing.

A home Scotch douche. A Scotch douche can perk you up more effectively than almost any other quick tonic bath. It requires a helper (with whom you can trade off for mutual benefit) and a couple of dollars' worth of extra equipment (which you can use over and over). However you'll find its extra benefits well worth the effort and expense.

Most fashionable watering places set aside a large room with special sprays and hoses for the Scotch douche, but you can get much the same results in the confines of your home as long as you have a shower stall and a sink in the same room. Here's how to do it:

> Clamp a shampoo spray unit (obtained from your drugstore or mail order house for less than two dollars) onto the sink faucet or faucets in your bathroom. Adjust your shower and shower curtain so that you can stand in a warm, continuous spray while your helper can squirt you with different temperature water from the shampoo unit. You can wear trunks or a brief bathing suit if modesty demands.
>
> After adjusting the shower to a comfortable warmth, you let it play upon your back and legs continuously throughout the first phase of the treatment. Your helper adjusts the stream from the shampoo unit into the HOT range, ideally 105 degrees measured with a candy or bath thermometer and definitely between 100 and 110 degrees. Holding the spray head close enough to make

impact give noticeable massage-like action, he should play the hot water stream up along your body from heel to calf to thigh, then up the spine, across to the shoulder and down the arm. Crossing the buttock area, he should start again at the opposite heel and play the stream up along a similar course again. Spraying both sides of the body should take twelve to forty seconds. Immediately after the HOT spray, your helper should shift to COLD water at about 65 degrees. If the undiluted cold water from the tap runs much colder than that in your part of the country (as it does here in Minnesota except in very late summer), he should leave a little dribble of hot coming through to take off the chill. He then plays the spray stream along the same course followed with the HOT water, but much more rapidly—three to ten seconds for both sides of the body. Repeat with the HOT, then with the COLD several times. Whenever you feel that you have had enough on your back, turn around and let your helper follow a similar routine on the front, avoiding only the genitals and abdomen. Turn again as desired, and continue for from three to ten minutes. Always end with a cold spray on your back for peak refreshment.

The cold friction bath. The cold friction bath is a quick refresher which works especially well when you feel exhausted from work or from the frantic evening rush of fixing dinner and setting the household in order. The more you're overheated, the better a cold friction bath works. So strip off your clothes while the bathtub fills and follow this procedure:

Adjust the bath temperature to between seventy and eighty degrees, which will feel cool rather than cold to your touch. Before getting into the tub, splash or pour some cold water over your head, face, neck and hands. Then quickly immerse your whole body up to the chin in the cool tub. You'll catch your breath with a gasp or two at first, but you'll soon breathe easy again. Rub the entire surface of your body briskly and continuously with both hands. You'll find that the friction makes you feel tolerably warm for from half a minute to three minutes. As soon as you begin to feel cold, get gooseflesh, or note a bluish tinge to your fingernails, get out of the tub and dry yourself quickly. Switch your wet towel for a dry, coarse one and rub all surfaces of your body with it briskly for one or two minutes.

As you become accustomed to cold friction baths, you'll be able to use somewhat cooler water and somewhat longer periods of immersion. The whole procedure never takes more than ten minutes, however, and it perks you up for literally hours.

Quick washcloth refresher. Although you need a bathroom method to bring on a complete tonic response, one quick and easy procedure which you can perform without taking off any clothing may refresh you considerably. When fatigue or dull routine begins to get you down, take sixty seconds to try this technique:

Lay a steaming hot washcloth—as hot as you can handle easily without risk of a burn—across the back of your neck for about thirty seconds. Use the still-warm cloth to scrub your face for a few seconds. End with several dashes of cold water on your cheeks and jowls, and towel yourself dry briskly.

TENSION-EASING BATHS AND APPLICATIONS

Racecourse living leaves almost everybody feeling tense at times. Even if tension doesn't pile up until it gives you a headache or other physical complaint, it makes every muscle in your body work harder and cuts down your energy reserve. That's why tension-fighting measures often prove even more refreshing than perk-up tonics, especially when you feel keyed up or nervously exhausted.

TENSION-SOOTHING OR TRANQUILIZING TUBS

A tranquilizing tub usually makes you feel distinctly unburdened and free of care. It lifts you "out of this world" as you float in water so close to your own skin temperature that you hardly know it is there, with just enough movement of fluid against your skin to reassure you that all is well. A wonderful mind-soothing retreat, effective against even the worst types of upheaval, which you can enjoy with virtually no trouble or expense. All you need is a bathtub and a thermometer. Here's the technique:

> Fill your tub partially with water between 92 and 94 degrees (or up to 96 degrees if the room is cool). Tie a washcloth or towel around the faucet in such a way that the water runs down along it instead of dribbling noisily. Adjust the water taps so that a steady, slight flow of lukewarm water continues, then get into the tub. Make yourself comfortable with a rolled towel underneath the back of your neck, and relax thoroughly. Check the water temperature at intervals, adjusting the taps to keep it in the proper range. Be sure the overflow drain works properly. Stay in the tub at least half an hour, and preferably about forty-five minutes. You will find that a feeling of quiet and torpor gradually suffuses your whole body, and that you feel marvelously calm. When ready to discontinue, dry yourself by wrapping your whole body in a bedsheet and patting the sheet against moist areas instead of by towel rubbing, which often disturbs your soothed feeling. Repeat with another sheet if necessary.

BRINE BATHS

When people first flocked to certain bathing places because of tonic or soothing effects, the spas depended on sea water. Natural brine has several advantages over fresh water for special baths:

it gives your body extra buoyancy, bestirs more circulation through your skin, and holds heat better. Even today, the Riviera, Bermuda and Hawaii—all warm sea-water bathing spots—mean tranquil ease and soothing relaxation to almost everyone, while mineral baths inland match the sea's restorative power mainly by mimicking its salt content.

You can enjoy the same effects in your own household if you so desire. Inexpensive water-softener salt works fairly well for most of the procedures, making supplies cost a few cents a bath. Your main expense stems from the fact that salt corrodes most metals and porcelain, so that a wooden tub, a plastic camper's tub or a reasonably deep child's wading pool works better than your normal bathroom fixtures. Most brine users bathe in the laundry room to use its water faucets and floor drain instead of rusting out their iron bathtub. Here's the detailed method:

> Put 8 to 10 pounds of salt in a few gallons of hot water at the bottom of the tub before you undress, so that it will have a chance to dissolve. When ready to bathe, add hot and cold water as needed to fill tub (about 40 gallons total) and adjust temperature to 94-98 degrees. If you use rock salt or other grit-containing varieties, let undissolved bits settle out and put a rubber bath mat over them before getting into the tub. During the bath, take a handful of table salt, let enough water run in to moisten it, and rub vigorously into the skin of your arms. Using additional salt if necessary, rub the legs, chest, abdomen and back. Avoid the sensitive tissues of the genitals and face, of course. Continue the salt rubbing until a pinkish glow suffuses your body surface, then lie back and relax in the tub for ten to fifteen minutes. Spray yourself with a shampoo unit (the easiest method in a laundry room) or length of hose to remove the salt as you get out of the tub, or take a quick shower bath. Dry off with brisk toweling after a daytime brine bath, or with sheets as described in conjunction with **tranquilizing tubs** if you plan to go right to sleep.

A few people prefer a solution which mimics sea water even more closely than plain salt solution. They use one pound of magnesium chloride and one-half pound of magnesium sulphate (both obtainable at any drugstore without prescription) for each tubful, in addition to the salt. This solution seems slightly more soothing to the skin, but makes the baths a bit more costly.

WASHROOM AND DESKSIDE SOOTHERS

A quick, tension-breaking refresher often keeps you calm and collected throughout a harried day when pressures would otherwise get you down. Simply breaking the pile-up of tension with a rest period helps, but a soothing water application doubles the benefit.

Hot face towels. At home, you can use the wringer or clothes-spinner on your washing machine to help you prepare a hot face towel. Soak the towel, or a piece of old flannel if you prefer, in hot water straight from the tap (140-180 degrees). Water at this temperature will burn your skin, so handle the towel with sticks or forceps. Put it through an ordinary wringer twice, or spin almost dry in your washing machine. Shake out trapped steam, which otherwise can cause burns. Lie down and drape the towel like a doughnut over your forehead, cheeks and chin, leaving the nose free for breathing. If the heat becomes too intense, lift the towel off for a few seconds, then replace it. DO NOT TRY TO USE THIS METHOD WITHOUT A WRINGER OR SPIN-DRY WASHER AT HAND. Water hot enough to do any good will burn both your hands and your face unless it is wrung out thoroughly.

Hot washcloths. If you work in an office or find yourself in need of tension-breaking refreshment when away from home, try the hot washcloth method. Without a wringer, use water no hotter than 112 degrees—moderately hot to the touch. Wring out the washcloth so that it will not drip, and apply to the back of your neck for about two minutes.

Soothing hand bath. An even easier tension-breaking refresher, especially apt before meals, involves use of hot cloths on the hands. Japanese restaurants have brought this wonderful custom over to this country, along with such innovations as shoes-off dining and table-side cookery. The steaming but well-wrung cloth comes to the table on a small wicker carrier. You can rub it gently between your palms, wipe along each of the fingers of first one hand and then the other, or simply hold it cupped between your hands while the relaxing warmth soothes your whole body. Try the same maneuvers in your own home: just wash your hands as usual, then run straight hot water on the washcloth, fold it between two layers of your towel and wring the towel and washcloth both together—a good way to get the excess moisture out of the cloth without burning your hands. Carry the washcloth to the table with you, and enjoy its soothing effects until you're ready to eat. Or try the same routine at deskside and between household chores. You'll be surprised at how much it perks you up.

Hot hand cloths probably refresh you because of nervous linkage between circulation of the hands and brain. Your hands and feet have special body-temperature-controlling circulation, which lets them detour blood to the cool skin surface or shunt it quickly through deep, warmth-holding passages. At least part of this action actually starts independently in the hands or feet, and apparently signals your brain to make adjustments in its own circulation. A hot foot bath thus clears your head, a warm hand cloth proves soothing, and many simple tonic applications to the hands and feet become very effective in altering the functions of the brain.

Foot baths. Some of the oldest tonics sometimes prove the best. Look to your Bible, for instance, to learn of Christ's own response to a foot bath. You can enjoy soothing and relaxing effect very similar to the long-acknowledged gentle bathing of your feet simply by dangling them in a tub, basin, or bucket filled partially with lukewarm water, and moving them back and forth slowly. Or you can use water flow through a shampoo spray tube to swirl warm water around your feet. Either technique proves very soothing, especially at the end of a long, hard day.

THIS CHAPTER'S SUGGESTIONS FOR USING WATER, A TOP-NOTCH REFRESHER AND TONIC

Water deserves some of the credit for the toned-up feeling you get from exercise and from other refreshers, besides doing noble work on its own. It can soothe or stimulate—make you feel literally "great"—by directly causing skin changes normally linked with emotion. The tonic response gives peak invigoration. Circulation spurred by exercise, massage or heat and followed by cold or friction usually brings on this response. Specific techniques include the tub-shower routine, the Scotch douche, and the cold friction bath. A less intense but still worthwhile perk-up response comes from the hot-washcloth-followed-by-cold-facebath routine, which you can perform in a minute or so without removing any clothes. If you need to calm down rather than perk up, try tranquilizing tubs, sea-water mimicking baths, hot facial towels, hot washcloths on your neck or hands, and foot baths.

Invigorating Rubdowns

Every race and nationality has a different way of getting ready for a big event. The typical German wants to know what's in store for him so that he can plan ahead for each detail. The typical Irishman wants to celebrate or drown his sorrows beforehand, while the typical Russian needs an interval of pessimistic lugubriation. But the Minnesota Swede has a unique approach. He doesn't try to cross his bridges either intellectually or emotionally before he comes to them. He simply tones up his body and mind so that he can meet whatever occurs efficiently and phlegmatically, usually with a program whose basic ingredient is massage. Massage calms your nerves, boosts your mood, tones up your muscles and clears cobwebs from your brain. What better preparation for either ordeal or beatitude?

SELF-ADMINISTERED MASSAGE

By adding chemical and friction-increasing action to the ordinary skin contact of message, you can get considerable tonic effect without fatiguing or tension-maintaining effort. For a self-administered, ten-to-fifteen minute home tonic that will put you "in the pink" in more ways than one, try the **salt glow.** You can expect such effects as:

> A vividly healthy-looking, pink, smooth skin.
> A feeling of fitness and rejuvenation.
> Measurable increase in your vigor and energy reserves.
> Improved circulation and elimination.

All in return for fifteen minutes or less of mild effort and about two pounds of ordinary table salt. The rest of the equipment can be found in almost any home, and is not damaged in any way by this procedure. You'll need:

1 one-quart basin or bowl
2 pounds table salt
2 bath towels
Shower, or bathtub equipped with shampoo-type hose and
    sprayhead.

A small wooden stool to sit upon inside the tub or shower also helps, but is not essential.

Preliminaries. Like most tonic procedures, the salt rub works best if you have been in a warm room (72 degrees or more) for two hours, or have been warmly dressed and well shielded from the elements. A hot tub for fifteen to thirty minutes beforehand also adds to the Salt Glow's effectiveness.

Salt makes metals rust, of course. If your tub or shower is finished with porcelain or tile, salt should cause no problems. A half inch of water in the bottom of the tub will dilute any drippings sufficiently to prevent rusting of the metal fittings around the plug, or you can coat metal parts with a bit of petroleum jelly. If you have a metal shower stall, best protect its bottom with a rubber sheet, a piece of plastic sheeting or a child's plastic wading pool until you are ready for your final rinse.

If you suffer from a skin rash other than pimples or from open sores, best omit Salt Glows unless your doctor gives you a go-ahead. Deep pimples of the back and chest usually benefit from Salt Glow massage, which would probably be widely used for adolescent rashes except for the fact that it cannot be applied to the soft-skinned face.

Preparation. Pour two pounds of table salt into a basin and break up any lumps. Add enough lukewarm water to form a paste-like sludge. Strip and get into the tub or shower stall, sitting on a small wooden stool if you have one available. Moisten your entire skin with lukewarm water unless you are still wet from a preliminary tub bath.

Procedure. Take some salt sludge in your right hand and begin the application on the back of the left wrist. Rub slowly in a circular fashion, using the palm of your hand rather than the fingers. Use firm pressure, but not enough to cause discomfort or injury. Eight to ten slow circuits in an area the size of your palm should suffice, then move up to the adjoining area. Continue to apply salt with definite friction, working your way up the arm to the shoulder and neck. Use somewhat gentler friction on the underside of the forearm and gentler still on the thin skin of the underside of the upper arm. Rub very softly or omit friction from the places where skin stretches over an underlying bony prominence.

Next, take some salt sludge in the left hand and apply in the same manner to the right wrist and arm.

Using both hands, work from the neck and shoulders down along the front of the trunk. Rub from side to side or along the rib lines in this area rather than using circular friction. Use a figure-eight motion around the breasts, avoiding the nipples.

Next, wet one of the bath towels and wring it out. Fold lengthwise until three or four layers thick. Spread a handful of salt sludge near the center of the towel. Lay the towel salted side down diagonally across your upper back, and grasp the two ends. Rub the salt into your shoulderblade area and upper chest with motions like those used to polish shoes. Apply moderate pressure, using eight to ten strokes in each area. After renewing the charge of salt, place the towel across your back in the opposite diagonal and do the areas previously missed. With another fresh charge of salt, place the towel across the small of your back and apply friction to the areas from shoulderblades to hips.

Start next at your ankles and work your way up, using both hands and applying salt with a rotary motion. Use firm pressure and ten to twelve strokes in each palm-sized area except over the anklebones and kneecaps, where heavy friction might cause injury. When you reach the inner thigh, try not to get salt on the genitals. If some salt does get into the reproductive organ's creases and folds, you will probably want to wash it free before it causes stinging and discomfort (although no permanent harm will be done).

Next, stand up. Take a handful of salt sludge in each hand. Rub into the buttock and hip areas with very strong rotary friction—the thick skin in these areas requires considerable pressure to call forth response.

Finally, finish off with a lukewarm shower or spray, and rub yourself down briskly with the remaining dry towel. Usually, you will find your skin soft and pink before the salt goes down the drain. A few people get a delayed reaction, with a pale skin for ten to fifteen minutes and a slowly developing pinkish glow thereafter. In any case, you'll usually feel simultaneously invigorated and relaxed long before you've completed a Salt Glow, and enjoy the effects for some time. Especially if followed by a period of exercise, a Salt Glow usually makes you feel better for several days, and two or three treatments a week won't do you a bit of harm.

Useful variations. If you take your salt rubs while seated on a stool in the bathtub, a simple variation makes them somewhat more effective. Simply put about six inches of moderately hot water (98 degrees measured with a candy thermometer) in the bottom of the tub and use it as a footbath. Gradually increase the temperature to 105 degrees by adding more hot water. Continue the footbath throughout the Salt Glow procedure. This increases circulation through the skin by reflex action, and supplements the response to salt and friction.

For a more powerful stimulation immediately after the treatment, simply use ice water rather than lukewarm water throughout the salt rub. Especially if combined with a preceding hot bath and continuing warm footbath, this makes the procedure extremely invigorating. Don't try the iced Salt Glow until you have become fast and certain at the ordinary variety, though. You must go quite fast and maintain fairly heavy friction to keep from getting chilled in the ice water variant, and it takes considerable practice to do this without risk of rubbing the skin raw over a bony prominence or in thinner areas.

Finally, you can give Salt Glows to other members of your family, and they can do the same for you, with tremendous effect. Cover a firm cot or table with plastic, oilcloth or rubber sheeting to avoid salt damage. Work from the ankles up to the thighs, from the wrists to the neck, down the front of the chest and then down the back to the hips and buttocks. Apply the salt and the friction with both hands, using rotary motions on the arms, legs, buttocks and lower back. Use strokes following the rib lines on the chest and figure-eight strokes around the breasts.

The Sponge Rub. An easier and more gentle form of self-administered massage is the Sponge Rub. Even people who cannot stand Salt Glow friction because of skin rashes or sore muscles and joints can often enjoy the sponge rub. It's an ideal soothing tonic for older people and convalescents. You should still check with your doctor before using this one if you have an open sore or severe eczema, but otherwise you can use this procedure whenever you're in good enough health for an ordinary tub bath.

You'll need the following equipment:

> One large plastic bath sponge with handle for reaching the back.
> Epsom salts, table salt and baking soda.
> Bathtub.

Be sure the room is warm and your body not unduly chilled. In a snugly stoppered bathtub, mix:

2 quarts lukewarm water.
4 ounces Epsom salts.
1 tablespoonful table salt.
1 tablespoonful baking soda.

Stir until the salts dissolve thoroughly. Undress, sit in the tub, and dip the sponge in solution. Rub the sopping sponge down the left arm from shoulder to fingers. Wet it again and sponge down the right arm. Sponge down your body from shoulders to hips in long vertical strokes, wetting the sponge thoroughly after each stroke. Sponge the thighs and legs, then attach the handle and sponge off your back. Continue rhythmic sponging for five to ten minutes. Drain off the solution. Sponge off thoroughly with several changes of cool water, gradually adjusting temperature downward. The final sponging should be with water at about 80 degrees, which will feel cool and refreshing but not cold. Fairly firm pressure and fairly vigorous strokes will create warming friction and let you use somewhat cooler water than you would otherwise tolerate without shivering or discomfort. Dry off with a bath towel or wrap yourself in a warm, dry sheet at the conclusion of the sponge rub.

Variations. When someone else administers a sponge rub for you, it may prove more invigorating if you use cold water rather than lukewarm to mix the original solution. Your helper can sponge more quickly and with firmer friction, which keeps the cool water from chilling your skin. Such cooler, friend-administered sponge rubs need last only three to five minutes. The effect is heightened if you dry off by wrapping in a sheet and letting your friend rub your entire body through the sheet with long, top-to-bottom strokes.

MOTOR-DRIVEN MASSAGE

Modern machines can do almost anything, from taking a fleck of soil off your white shirt to gouging a ton at a time out of the earth. Most machines let you do things you otherwise couldn't accomplish or make an otherwise wearisome job somewhat easier. Massage machines do both, but with somewhat limited success.

Vibrating tables or chairs. While collecting material for this book, I asked one of my colleagues how he managed to last through his ten-to-twelve-hour days without any trace of wilt.

"Sit in that leather chair over there and I'll show you," he said.

A push and a pull on the chair revealed a footrest and collapsed the back into lounging position. The click of a switch started a gentle, all-over vibration.

"Just relax in that chair for a few minutes," my colleague said. "You'll feel like a new man. That's what I do for five minutes every hour I'm in the office. Keeps me fresh as a daisy from morning till night."

Perhaps five minutes of relaxation every hour would have kept my friend refreshed whether his chair vibrated or not. The soothing drone of the vibrator motor might have had as much to do with the chair's effect as its action. Whatever the explanation, some people find such chairs and tables quite refreshing.

Motor-driven hand vibrators. A small, inexpensive vibrator motor which attaches to the back of your hand lets you administer some forms of massage to yourself. It also aids any member of your family who volunteers as your masseur.

The big advantage in a vibrator is its effort-sparing action: it lets you give yourself massage and simultaneously relax, or lets a person whose muscles would grow weary from kneading or pounding give you a vigorous rubdown. These benefits often make a vibrator worth its moderate price, even though you get no effect from it which a good masseur cannot get with his hands alone.

Tension-breaking massage of the head, neck and shoulders usually proves to be the most useful form of self-administered vibrator massage. Be sure your fingernails are well trimmed, or cover them with a cotton work glove. With the vibrator on the back of your hand, hold your fingers limp and relaxed as you rub them slowly from eyebrows to nape in rhythmic strokes. Press the fingers loosely into tense face muscles, moving them in slow spirals over the lips, cheeks and brow. Press the flat of your hand against tight muscles at the back and sides of your neck for stronger action than the limp fingers will transmit, or knead these muscles with your whole hand while simultaneously letting the vibrator run.

Several of my patients also use a hand vibrator for the sake of more attractive hair and skin. Scalp massage with a vibrator increases the flow of natural oil and helps to spread it along the hair shafts, often doing away with the need for artificial hair-dressings and giving the hair an attractive natural sheen. It may improve dry, flaky dandruff considerably. Facial skin may also improve in texture from vibrator massage if lack of natural oils is at fault. No form of massage effectively combats baldness or wrinkles, however.

If you can get one of your family or friends to give you a rub-down, a vibrator works very well on the muscle masses of your back, arms and legs. After vigorous exercise or fatiguing work, a thorough rubdown proves very refreshing. Vibrator-aided massage also tones up flabby muscles after inactivity or illness, and relaxes accumulated tension. For gentle massage, your helper keeps his fingers loose as he presses them into the muscles. He simultaneously moves his hands in slow, lengthwise ovals along each part. Fingernails should be well-trimmed, or a household rubber glove used to pad them. Mineral oil works well as a lubricant.

Clean it off afterward with rubbing alcohol and two or three
hand towels. Use talcum powder as a lubricant if you wear a
rubber glove, since oil ultimately rots rubber. Or you can use
camphor and soap liniment, U.S.P., available in any pharmacy
without prescription. A steady, rhythmic motion with gradually
heavier vibration obtained by stiffening the fingers works best.
Tight shoulder and neck muscles may respond well to grasping or
kneading with the vibrator-agitated hand. Tight muscles along
the sides of the spinal column usually feel better if the knuckles
of a vibrating fist are pressed into them in one place after another
and worked in a rotary fashion within the range of skin elasticity.
A slow buildup in intensity of massage followed by a fairly slow
tapering to gentle, lax-finger action leaves you feeling soothed
and greatly refreshed.

TURN-AND-TURN-ABOUT MASSAGE

From watching the monkeys in the zoo, I've concluded that
one principle dates back farther than the human race, namely:
"You scratch my back and I'll scratch yours." So it doesn't seem
too far-fetched that two human members of the same family might
willingly use the same kind of turn-and-turn-about with slightly
more gentle frictions, and give each other tonic massage.

The drip sheet bath. You can get substantial soothing and
tonic effects from unskilled massage through a wet sheet. Vigor
counts for more than experience in giving this rubdown. If your
helper can reach every part of your body easily without strain
and works willingly at his task, you'll almost certainly get good
results.

For a drip sheet bath, you need:

> 2 sheets
> 3 buckets or waterproof plastic wastebaskets
> Candy or bath thermometer

Small stool
Mat to improve footing if required
Bathroom with washbasin and tub or shower.

Preliminaries: Your helper can wear a bathing suit or other outfit which will not be harmed by water. You should either undress completely (which gives best results) or strip down to brief underpants. Your response will be best if your body is thoroughly warm from at least two preceding hours in a comfortably heated room (72 degrees or more). Many people get extra effects if they take a hot footbath before or during the rubdown—water well above the ankles, starting at about 98 degrees and adding hot water gradually until it reaches 105.

Before your first drip sheet bath, you should go through several dry runs with your helper to master the art of getting into the sheet quickly. Your helper holds the sheet, which has been unfolded and gathered from one end like a drawn curtain, while you raise your arms. Your helper puts the upper corner of the sheet in your right armpit. You lower your right arm to hold it in place, and turn to your right. The sheet wraps around your body under your left arm and across your back. Drop your left arm, and turn further until the sheet is wrapped around your entire body. Your helper tucks the upper corner of the sheet snugly in at the neck or pins it in place, and loosely presses some of the loose sheeting between your legs to separate them. If you have wrapped correctly no two skin surfaces meet without a layer of sheeting between them. When you can achieve this result quickly and surely with a dry sheet, you can proceed.

Preparation: Warm one of the sheets in an oven or on a radiator. Unfold the other, and gather it in folds from one end like an open window-drape. Partially fill your washbasin with water at 75-80 degrees, and immerse the gathered sheet into it. Place the stool in the bathtub or at the entrance to your shower stall so that your helper can sit down while massaging your body from shoulders to knees. Fill the three buckets with water slightly colder than that used to soak the wet sheet—the first about two degrees colder, the next about four degrees colder, and the third about six degrees colder. Now wring out the wet sheet partially, just enough so that it can be handled easily.

Procedure: Wrap yourself quickly in the cool, wet sheet. As soon as it is securely fastened in place, have your helper sit on the stool and massage you vigorously through the sheet with both hands. He should take long, top-to-bottom strokes down your back, arms, front and legs as far as the knees, turning you as necessary. Occasionally, he varies the massage by giving a succession of slaps running down the back and buttocks or arms and legs.

Massage and slapping quickly draw warm blood to the skin surfaces. Your helper will feel body warmth through the wet sheet when this happens. If some areas warm up before others, he should concentrate a bit more attention on the lagging areas until the sheet has warmed over your entire body surface. Between two and ten minutes are required to reach this stage, depending on the vigor of your helper's efforts and of your skin's reaction. If you continue to feel chilly and show no signs of skin reaction after three to five minutes, the chances are that your helper did not work quickly or vigorously enough. You will not get a good reaction if it has not started by this time, so you should unwind the sheet, take a warm shower, and try again some other day. If you still fail to react well, you are probably one of the few who respond poorly to this kind of massage, and should use other tonic techniques instead.

When your helper feels the warmth of your skin penetrating through the sheet all over, he empties the warmest pail of water over your head, shoulders and trunk. He immediately begins to stroke and slap again through the sopping-wet sheet. You usually can take more vigorous rubbing and slapping at this stage than at first, and your skin warms much more quickly. When body warmth penetrates all over the sheet again, your helper pours the second warmest pail over your head, shoulders and trunk, and once more rubs and slaps through the dripping sheet. The third and coolest pail follows when warmth has been restored, again with vigorous massage. When the skin has thoroughly warmed after the final pail, you should get out of the wet sheet and quickly wrap up in the warm, dry one, using the same wrapping technique as before. Your helper rubs you down with vigorous, top-to-bottom strokes through the sheet until your skin is thoroughly dry. At this point you should feel somewhat fatigued but greatly soothed and refreshed. Your skin should have a uniform, pinkish glow. After a fifteen to thirty minute rest, you should feel literally "great."

When your skin has become accustomed to react and your helper has become more skilled, you can gradually lower the temperature of the water used for drip sheet baths. Keep the successive stages—sheet soak and three pails—each about two degrees cooler than its predecessor, and lower the sheet soak's temperature about two or three degrees with each application until you reach the upper sixties. You'll find drip sheet baths more and more refreshing and invigorating as the temperature cools.

The moist sheet bath. If you need a quicker and less fatiguing home rubdown, or if you want a perk-up routine that leaves you ready to go without a preliminary period of rest, the moist sheet bath probably will suit you perfectly. Warm one sheet in an oven or on a radiator. Unfold another, gather it from the end like a drawn drape, and soak in water at 60-80 degrees —near 60 if you are accustomed to drip sheet baths or hot-cold showers, near 80 if you haven't built skin reactivity. Wring out the sheet very thoroughly with the aid of your helper. Now wrap yourself in the moist sheet as described in the last section, and have your helper rub you vigorously with both hands, using top-to-bottom strokes from shoulder to knee level and from the front, back and sides. The slapping motions advised with a dripping-wet sheet are too harsh with a moist one, and should not be used. When your entire skin feels warm through the sheet, discard the moist sheet and replace with the dry one. Have your helper rub further with long, top-to-bottom strokes until you are entirely dry. This procedure takes only five to ten minutes, including time to set up and restore order. It generally leaves you feeling greatly refreshed and invigorated.

The tension- and fatigue-soothing backrub. A shower and a rubdown after a day's work often turns weariness into a relaxed glow. Nervous tension yields to similar measures, such as a warm, relaxed tub followed by slow-paced, soothing backrub. Even the dull, fuzzy feeling you suffer from boredom and the creaks and cricks of unusual inactivity pass off after a few minutes of rhythmic stroking.

Backrubs require more skill than sheet baths. You can easily learn to give them, though, by following these suggestions:

Trim your fingernails. The slightest scratching at the end of each stroke kills its soothing action. Even with short nails, you'll need to remain constantly alert to this problem. Long nails make scratching almost inevitable.

Provide ease and comfort. Loose clothing and convenient arrangements make it much easier to give a smooth, effective backrub. Working height is especially important: if you have to bend over to reach certain parts of the back, your muscles will be tense and your motions jerky. Often you will find it easier to pad a table than to give massage in an ordinary bed. Or you can raise each end of the bed by placing its bottom rail on the seats of one or two straight chairs.

Use lotion, oil or shortening for lubrication. Backrub lotions, of which most drugstores carry several sorts, cost very little and help in several ways. If your hands are the least bit rough or calloused, lotion makes them feel more smooth. In winter weather, lotion helps to fight dryness. And you can give a backrub without clipping thick body hair if you use a lubricating product, but usually cannot do so with ordinary alcohol. If lotions seem too expensive, try baby oil, light salad oil, or an odorless vegetable shortening such as Crisco.

Stroke evenly. Rhythm makes a backrub much more soothing: rhythm in the strokes and rhythm in the pauses. Swaying your body slightly with each stroke usually gives your backrub just the smoothness they need. If you place one foot a little in front of the other, you can lean into each stroke, lift your hands and lean backward, then place your hands against the back and stroke forward again in perfect rhythm.

Use your palms, not your fingertips. Fingertips dig in, and fingernails scratch. Keep your hands flat, with the fingers fairly well relaxed but close together.

Blend into the pressure phase of each stroke, and then out of it again. Pressure should be quite light throughout each stroke at the beginning. Later, as you warm to the task and the back muscles begin to relax, you can increase pressure near the center of each stroke. Pressure should be extremely light at the beginning and end of each stroke. Light touch firming to gentle pressure then tapering to light touch again makes a perfect movement. During the last few minutes, you should taper to gentle touch again.

Make all your strokes in the same direction. Start your backrubs by placing both hands beside the base of the spine, stroking gently up toward the base of the neck, then curving out toward the shoulders at the upper end of your reach. Lift the hands, bring them back to almost the same spot at which you started the previous stroke, and carry the next one along practically the identical course. Work your way gradually up the back. When your strokes reach the muscle masses at the base of the neck, grasp them between your joined fingers and the heel of your hand, then stroke along them toward the point of the shoulders. When your strokes begin between the shoulder blades, it is time to work your way back down the back and start over. To do this, make your hands into fists and press the second-joint knuckles into the muscle masses beside the upper spine. Move the pressed-in knuckles up and down several times along the course of the spinal column within the range of the skin's elasticity, going as far as possible without sliding along the skin. Lift the knuckles, place them an inch or two farther down the back, and repeat. Move to the base of the spine in this way, then start open-hand massage with upward strokes again.

End with alcohol, light toweling and talcum powder. Near the end of your backrub, let all of the lotion or shortening soak into the skin. Switch to rubbing alcohol for the final, light-stroke phase. If the back feels greasy, dry off the first batch of alcohol with a hand towel and apply once more. Finally, dry off the back and powder lightly with talcum.

A backrub feels wonderful when you come home tired or tense. And it's a fine form of turn-and-turn-about massage: you don't need to rest or exercise afterwards, so you can go straight from being rubbed to rubbing. For peak effect on fatigue, take your backrub after a hot-cold shower. For peak effect on nervous tension use the backrub after a soothing warm tub. But use this procedure often: you'll find it a fine refresher.

All-over massage. In posh businessman's clubs, in big-time athletic locker rooms, in the highest-priced luxury resorts—wherever cost counts less than effectiveness—massage reigns supreme as a tonic and refresher. All but a few people react splendidly to it: feel new verve and keenness for literally days. You can enjoy new vigor, a great lift in mood, and quick relief from tension or fatigue from all-over massage, whether administered by a professional or performed by a friend or member of the family. Anyone who has learned to give a good backrub can perform an adequate all-over massage. The position, the strokes and the rhythm are the same. Only the parts rubbed differ.

Before starting massage, review the section on backrubs point by point. Fingernails trimmed? Comfortable clothing and arrangements? Lotion or lubricant available? Ready to make your strokes even in rhythm, with palms rather than fingertips, beginning and ending quite lightly, and all strokes in the same direction? Alcohol, towels and talcum powder on hand for a windup?

Now uncover one of the subject's legs completely, being sure that no tight clothing at the thigh or groin cuts down free circulation. Prop the lower leg up on two or three pillows, roughly parallel with the floor—if you prop the heel much higher than the thigh, the muscle cords at the back of the knee slow down circulation through deep-lying veins. Begin with long, even strokes starting at the knee and running to the hip, rubbing both hands along the front and sides of the thigh. Keep strokes long, steady and even, maintaining rhythm even when your hands are not in contact with the skin. Work gradually down to the ankle. Take about five minutes to finish the leg, then wipe off any excess lotion or lubricant, and cover to maintain warmth.

Move next to the corresponding arm. Prop it up on one or two pillows, and start massage with strokes from elbow to shoulder. Work gradually down the arm to the wrist. Move the subject to the other side of the bed. Massage the opposite leg and arm, taking about five minutes for each extremity. Then turn him over on his abdomen and massage each leg from calf to upper thigh, taking about five minutes apiece. Cover the legs and finish with a thorough backrub, which takes another fifteen minutes for a forty-five minute total. Use rubbing alcohol and talcum powder on the back and on any parts which still seem oily to touch, and let the subject rest for about half an hour.

This form of massage, in which waste products and stagnant blood are milked out of every vein and muscle into previously-cleared-out areas, works especially well for relieving fatigue and increasing vigor. Even one such rubdown a week usually makes a big difference to the way you feel, especially if performed after a hot tub, steam bath or good workout. When nervous tension seems more of a problem than physical vigor, you usually get better results with exactly the opposite routine: backrub before extremities, stroking down the arms and legs instead of up them, doing the back of the extremities before the front. Such outward-moving massage seems to drive away troubles, and gives great relief for tension and blue mood.

CHAPTER TWO'S REFRESHING RUBDOWNS

Massage calms your nerves, boosts your mood, tones up your muscles and clears cobwebs from your brain. You can enjoy self-administered, mechanical, or turn-and-turn-about varieties of massage at home without undue expense.

A *salt glow* should make you look and feel much more vigorous and fit, besides combatting body pimples. A simultaneous hot footbath or ice-cold water rather than lukewarm in your salt mixture increases the effect. The *sponge rub* gives similar benefits with a gentler and easier routine, especially beneficial for older people and convalescents.

Motorized massage with vibrating chairs or tables seems refreshing to some people. A hand vibrator lets you give yourself some forms of massage while still relaxing sufficiently to get some good out of them, and lets untrained members of your family give massage without becoming fatigued. Self-administered massage of the head, neck and shoulders usually relaxes accumulated tensions after a wearing day. Scalp and facial massage may improve appearance somewhat, too. Friend-administered massage of the back, arms and legs proves very refreshing after vigorous work or play, helps to relax your accumulated tensions, and tones up flabby muscles after illness or inactivity.

If a friend or member of your family will undertake to give you a massage, a drip sheet bath calls for very little skill and gives substantial soothing and tonic effects. A quick and easy variant is the moist sheet bath, which perks you up in ten minutes or less. Backrubs work especially well for soothing tension and fatigue. All-over massage gives new vigor, a great lift in mood and quick relief from tension or fatigue, and is easily learned by anyone who has mastered the backrub. If you aim to relieve fatigue and increase physical vigor, massage toward the heart. If you aim to ease blue moods and nervousness, massage outward along the various body parts.

CHAPTER THREE

Soothing and Tonic Rays

Most of my winter-vacationer patients bring back the same story from Florida or California:

"A few hours on the beach bakes new strength and vigor into my muscles," they say. "Not to mention extra suppleness into my joints and contentment into my soul."

Maybe the effect seems greater when you haven't enjoyed Old Sol for several months and chase his favors full time. But you can get a lot of benefit from the sun right in your own back yard. Sunlamps or bakers can give you lots of help, too, whether natural sunshine is available or not.

SUNBATHING

In Minneapolis, the worst jam of the year usually ties up lakeshore traffic on the first warm day of May. The water itself remains too cold for bathing until late June, but the grassy lakeside slopes nearly disappear beneath sunbathers' blankets, and the roads fill bumper-to-bumper with creeping cars. Sunbathing is a serious business for most of these people, too, and not just an excuse for flirting and bodily display. You'll often see three generations of Swansons or Olsons stretched out on adjoining patches. Middle-aged and old folks who come to soak up the healing, invigorating rays often outnumber the young adults and children, in spite of the fact that they spend only a few minutes basking in the world's most ancient tonic, then go their way.

A few get *more* than they bargain for. Winter pallor makes your skin burn all too readily, and prolonged sun exposure also involves other risks. However, you can benefit from the sun's tonic action entirely without damage by following a few simple rules:

1. Expose yourself GRADUALLY. If you're dead pale after a sunless winter, and especially if your complexion is very fair, start off with skyshine instead of direct sun. Five minutes of noonday exposure in open shade may ultimately pinken a fair skin. An increase to ten, fifteen and twenty minutes on successive days makes a very suitable preliminary. When you start sunning yourself directly, lie always on your back with your face well protected. Keep your upper body in open shade and expose only your feet on the first day. The thick foot-skin can almost always stand five full minutes of noon sun, while an initial five-minute exposure often burns the torso. On the second sunning, you can give your feet five minutes, then move a bit farther out of the shade to include your lower legs for an additional five minutes. In this way, your feet get ten minutes of direct sun while your legs get only five. On the next sunning, give your feet five minutes, your feet and lower legs another five, and your whole legs another five for fifteen minutes total. The next day, follow this routine with five minutes' exposure of your body from the waist down. The next day add five minutes for the entire body, so that your feet get 25 minutes, your lower legs 20, your thighs 15, your lower trunk 10, and your chest 5. The next day add five minutes lying on your stomach to expose your back, and then increase each interval slightly to prolong exposure bit by bit. In about two weeks, you will have a good enough tan to tolerate all-over sun exposure for half an hour, and that is all you really need for tonic effect.

If part by part increase in sunning seems too complicated, you can simply cut back all your sun exposure to match the slowest-tanning areas. After preliminary periods in open shade, start with a two minute sunbath and work up two minutes at a time. You'll get a tan much more slowly, especially on your legs, but you won't suffer sunburn in the process.

2. Protect your face from direct sunshine. The thin skin of your face burns easily, dries out with excessive sun, and gets enough excess exposure during your lifetime to set off an occasional abnormal growth. You cannot increase the tonic effects of sunbathing appreciably by exposing your face, which involves a very small proportion of your body surface. Rather than risk harmful effects, protect your head with a suitable hat or parasol.

3. Adjust for time and season. Many Minnesotans begin the sunning season in the late afternoon, after work or school. Maybe they build up to an hour or more exposure without harmful effects. Then comes a clear weekend, and many people sun themselves for the same period at midday. Painful sunburn almost always results. Reason: the sun has four times as much burning power at midday as at 5:30.

You can figure the approximate strength of sun rays at different times of day from this table: *

Time of Day (Standard, Not DST)	Strength of Sun Compared with Midday
6 a.m.	1/5
7 a.m.	2/5
8 a.m.	3/5
9 a.m.	3/4
10 a.m.	9/10
11 a.m.	
12 noon	Approximately equal
1 p.m.	
2 p.m.	9/10
3 p.m.	3/4
4 p.m.	3/5
5 p.m.	2/5
6 p.m.	1/5

* Total sunlight falling on a horizontal surface on a clear midsummer day in the Midwest, adapted from *Applications of Germicidal, Erythemal and Infrared Energy,* Matthew Luckeish, D.Sc., D.E., D. Van Nostrand Company, Inc., New York 1946. Differences are slightly less in southern climes.

In other words, if you know you can spend an hour in the sun at 6 p.m., best keep to 1/5 that time, or 12 minutes, at midday. Or *vice versa*—if you've worked up to ten minutes of midday sun, you can tolerate five times as much (or 50 minutes) after 6 o'clock standard time.

4. *Ignore warmness in setting exposure times.* The sun's warming rays are long infrared rays which pass through the atmosphere at any angle. The rays responsible for tanning and for sunburn filter out as they pass through air. They are much stronger at noon when the sunlight passes straight down through the atmosphere than in the late afternoon when it strikes at an angle and must pass obliquely through the earth's air blanket. Suntan rays are stronger in the mountains for the same reason: a mountain climber or skier has less air between him and the sun, and thus may get sunburned in much less time than at sea level.

When the sun's warmth seems slight, as on a cool, overcast day, few infrared rays reach your skin. But the ultraviolet rays, which cause both tanning and burn, may still be very strong. Sunbathers have to keep this fact in mind so that they will not burn themselves when the sun does not seem strong or hot.

5. *Let* LATE *reaction guide your sun exposure.* If you stay out in the sun on a warm day, your skin will turn somewhat pink. A lot of people think this pinkness is an early warning that sunburn may result from longer exposure, and continue to sun themselves until it appears. Actually, immediate pinkness comes from the sun's infrared rays, not from its sunburn-causing ultraviolet. On a slightly overcast day, you can get a severe sunburn without any immediate pinkness at all. You must wait at least twelve hours to judge your reaction to a given amount of sunlight. If you get even slight, long-delayed redness, decrease future planned exposures somewhat. If no redness develops, you can increase exposure on schedule.

6. *Use suntan oils for sunburn protection, not tanning aid.*

Suntan preparations act as sunray filters, letting through only a small portion of the ultraviolet light which strikes them. You can stay out in the sun about seven times as long if you coat your skin with suntan oil. However, it takes almost seven times as long to get a suntan, too. Tanning preparations don't usually help you to get a better tan: they just help you to keep from burning yourself if you spend time in the sun before tanning is complete.

7. Shield prominences from excessive exposure. No matter how tanned you become, excessive sun exposure may cause peeling on your shoulders, nose, and forehead. Petroleum jelly gives good protection from such changes. Dark amber or orange-red jelly works best—the darker the better. A very thin layer on heavy exposure areas cuts sunburn rays to 1/20th of their previous strength.

8. Take precautions against excess heat. When the mercury hovers above eighty, sunbathing can prove a warm sport. Even when the breezes blow, your body has to put out extra salt-containing sweat to keep your temperature at its proper level. When you expose yourself for a long time, you should therefore take extra salt. Either salt tablets or heavily-salted foods help. If you get signs of heat fatigue, such as dizziness, extreme exhaustion or nausea, always get out of the sun promptly. Be especially careful to protect your head from sun on warm days, too.

If you follow these eight rules, the summer sun should add a good deal to your vigor and tranquility. A few minutes three or four times a week will give good effect. Longer or more frequent sessions may give some further benefit, but usually not enough to prove worthwhile.

SUNNING IN WINTERTIME

You can benefit somewhat from the sun's tonic rays even during the cold months if you have a window, skylight or door so situated that you can sunbathe beneath it. A pane of glass blocks off the sun's beneficial rays completely, however: you have to cover a window screen or screen door with thin, clear plastic to make a sun-admitting portal. Even with this procedure, sunlight gives relatively weak rays in wintertime: in the northern U.S.A., December and January sun has only one-fourth the tanning power of summer sun, while late fall and early spring rays have about half their summer strength. At that, the sun remains as strong a source of tonic rays as most inexpensive sunlamps. Unless a cloudy climate or a crowded daytime schedule makes it unavailable, twenty or thirty minutes' exposure about three times a week will give you considerable benefit. Rig a plastic-covered sun window and use it between ten and two if you live in the midwest, or between nine and three in the southern climes.

If the midday hour or a plastic-protected sunbathing window won't work out for you, ultraviolet baths might prove worthwhile. Most of the sun's skin-toning action comes from ultraviolet. If you have a pimply complexion or skin blemishes which clear in summertime, you will probably get the same benefits from ultraviolet as from true sunbaths. Since glass blocks skin-toning ultraviolet rays, you need to use a quartz type generator. In larger cities, you can test your response by renting a lamp, joining a health club, or arranging a series of sunbaths in the physiotherapy department of your doctor's favorite hospital. Or you can buy a small generator for your home. If you buy, get a quartz-tube mercury arc lamp rather than a screw-in bulb. The shorter time needed for each sunbath and greater effectiveness make its somewhat high cost worthwhile.

CABINET BODY BAKER BATHS

Walk into any luxurious businessman's club, and you'll find a well-patronized department devoted to Turkish baths. A few of the customers will be fighting hangover, but most of them simply want to feel "great" and work more efficiently.

In the training room of any big league team—football, base-
ball, basketball or hockey—you'll find players baking joints
or muscles under a heat lamp. Sometimes they're treating sprains
or strains, but quite often they're trying to bake a little extra
limberness into an aging part.

You can combine both kinds of action, and stimulate sluggish
circulation, too, with an inexpensive, homemade body baker.
You'll need:

> 3 300 watt lightbulbs in metal reflectors
> 3 screw eyes
> string or cord
> a blanket
> some safety pins
> a few pincer clothespins
> a wooden or metal chair or stool without inflammable
> plastic upholstery

Choose a convenient bedroom corner and drive screw eyes into
the wall three feet from the floor at the corner and four feet along
each of the two walls. Place your chair in the corner, facing toward the room. Place the three floodlamps in the corner and at
each side of the chair so that they form a triangle around it. Run
a piece of cord across the corner between the two side-wall screw
eyes. Fasten two adjacent corners of the blanket to the screw eye
in the room's corner. The slack edge between these attached corners becomes a head hole just above the chair or stool. Use safety
pins to close the unneeded part of the opening.

Always use your body baker with someone else in the room or
within call, to give aid in the one-in-a-thousand instance of dizziness or fainting. This reaction occurs when over-brisk response
detours too much blood to the skin and leaves the brain without
enough circulation. It clears up promptly if you get your head
down between your knees or lie down, but you may need help to
get out of the apparatus.

Take body baker baths only after you have been in a fairly warm room—72 degrees, or more—for at least two hours. Recent chilling will keep down your skin's reaction.

Strip and sit on the stool, facing toward the middle of the room. Turn on the lights. Pass your head through the head hole and drape the blanket over the diagonal cord so that it encloses your body and all three lamps. Use clothespins to hold the blanket in place if necessary. Be sure that it does not come into contact with the hot lamps. The soothing rays and accumulating heat will usually put you into a definite sweat inside ten minutes.

When your skin is moist and rosy-pink, turn off the lamps and go directly to your shower stall. Start with warm water, but adjust it quickly to colder and colder temperatures, rubbing briskly with both hands in the areas where the water strikes. You will gasp momentarily as cold water strikes each new body area, but the floods of warming blood which the ray bath has brought to your skin soon make the shower feel almost like warm syrup. Continue to adjust the temperature colder and colder until you have reached a low temperature and showered in it for ten to thirty seconds. Quit the moment you begin to feel cold, and dry yourself thoroughly with a warm towel. Switch to a dry towel and rub yourself briskly all over for an additional sixty seconds. You'll feel totally clean, as if you had scrubbed clear down into your pores, and greatly refreshed and invigorated. The hot air bath and shower make a tonic as strong as any Turkish bath in town, while the penetrating infrared and visible rays that saturate your whole body surface in the light cabinet boost sluggish circulation and do wonders for stiff muscles or joints.

You shouldn't take body-baker baths if you have heart trouble, skin trouble which perspiration aggravates, or joints which are red and swollen from any form of arthritis. You should omit the cold shower phase if you have trouble with high blood pressure, poor circulation or chilblains. Otherwise, you'll get a lot of benefit from this tonic routine.

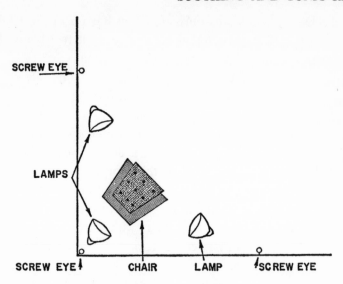

"HEAT LAMPS" AND HEATING PADS

You can get a lot of benefit from heat rays both in toning up circulation and in restoring yourself after overexertion. You needn't waste money on a special "heat lamp," either: the rays from an ordinary 300 watt bulb penetrate as deep as those from any heat lamp, and do just as much good.

Lightbulb heat as a circulation booster. You should never heat blood-starved tissue, whether poor circulation, cold exposure * or prolonged, cramped sitting is at fault. Heat increases need for fuel more quickly than it improves poor circulation. It can cause temporary pain or even lasting damage. However, lightbulb heat boosts circulation safely if you use it to warm the blood *on its way* to the affected part. Warming rays on your hips and upper thighs (preferably from the front, where the main blood vessels run near the surface) will speed up circulation in your legs and feet. Warming rays shining on the base of your

---

* The one exception is in thawing true frostbite, where circulation must be restored at any price.

neck and shoulder or into your armpit increase blood flow in the affected arm and hand. Faster circulation carries away fatigue-causing acids and rebuilds reserve-strength fuel deposits in your muscles. It chases the chill from half-frozen hands and feet. Warm blood eases pins-and-needles feeling and coldness due to sluggish circulation. Yet the parts themselves remain cool until enough blood has reached them.

Lightbulb heat after overexertion. Here in Minnesota, you're always likely to find yourself having to overexert. Like the time my wife's car slid off the packed snow in our driveway into a three-foot-high drift. It took me nearly an hour with the snow shovel and some arduous pushing, plus the old trick of pushing the car off the jack, to get her back on the track. That's a lot of work for a soft desk worker! But I didn't have a stiff muscle in my body, thanks to lightbulb heat. A 300 watt bulb in a metal floodlight reflector burning about 18 inches away from my bared back soothed the strained muscles before they got a chance to ache.

You can use this same approach after almost any kind of muscular over-indulgence. Bake new energy into your bowling arm, your golfer's shoulder, or your snowshoveler's back before stiffness has time to get a start. Twenty to thirty minutes of light-bulb heat while you're reading the newspaper or watching TV almost always restores over-used muscles to total suppleness.

Lightbulb heat in sexual congestion. A lot of home reme-dies work on the principle that blood can't flow in two directions at once. Hot foot baths relieve a cold's congested nose, Turkish baths or body-baker baths detour blood away from the brain to ease congestion-type hangover headaches. You can apply the same idea to fight sexual congestion.

A number of unpleasant sensations and sexual weaknesses stem from pooling of blood in the sex organs: masculine dis-comfort and poor performance after a period without fulfillment, physical and emotional troubles which plague both men and women when thorough arousal is not followed by a satisfying climax, and so on. Many men who have endured countless treatments for "boggy prostate" or "low-grade prostatitis" also suffer from nothing more or less than sexual congestion.

You get no relief from heating the sexual organs themselves in any of these conditions. The crucial blood vessels lie too deep within your tissues. But you can often get considerable relief by lying in a position which helps blood drain away from the sex organs, then opening up blood vessels in other body parts through use of heat. Lie on your stomach with three or four pillows under your hips and with one or two 300 watt bulbs shining from a distance of 12 to 18 inches on both your legs and your upper back. As the exposed skin surfaces turn distinctly pink from extra flow of blood, you will usually feel considerable relief of your sexual congestion. If the warm rays to other parts do not suffice, however, a padded ice bag or cold, wet, folded towel in the crotch area increases the effect.

Menstrual cramps and discomfort sometimes stem from similar circulatory stagnation, and yield to the hips-high, warmed-legs-and-trunk system. Cold applications increase cramping, however, and should not be used.

Heating pads. A heating pad gives warmth by generating rays, not by direct heat flow. In fact, its blanket-like outer lining cuts out almost all direct heat transfer. A heating pad has no real advantage over lightbulb or heat lamp heat except ease of application, and has several disadvantages. Most heating pads have "hot spots" which become ten degrees or more warmer than the rest of the pad. To keep these hot spots from burning, you need to set the temperature considerably lower than you would tolerate with evenly distributed lightbulb heat. You can't regulate the heat you get from them as easily as that from a lamp, which can be moved closer or farther to give exactly the heat you desire. In fact, you may find only one temperature setting really usable— most pads can cause burns, especially on parts with poor circulation, when set either "medium" or "high," leaving only the "low" setting available. And heating pads cost much more than light-bulbs.

Still, you may find a heating pad more convenient than a lamp when your circulation needs a boost or when you have over-exerted yourself. You can use a pad without shedding all your clothes, which often lets you apply heat when you wouldn't other-wise take the trouble. If you decide on this technique, use the low heat setting, never put a blanket or sweater on top of the pad or put the element under your body, and never apply heat directly to chilled or circulation-starved parts. With these precautions, you can safely get benefit from a heating pad without spending hardly any time or effort.

"SUCKER"-SWINDLING RAYS

From cosmic ray emanators to radiation caves, hundreds of invisible "healing" rays have been foisted on the public by swin-dlers. Literally millions of dollars every year go to charlatans who take advantage of the fact that faith in their spiel can half-hypnotize perfectly normal and wise people into feeling tem-porary improvement.

It is true that you cannot see or feel every ray that might bene-fit you—X-rays and true ultraviolet, for example. But it is also true that a telephone call to your local Better Business Bureau or to your family doctor might save you a lot of ray-emanator money. Before you put cash into any you-can't-see-it-but-it's-there health booster, make sure that you're dealing with a totally honest individual.

SOOTHING AND TONIC RAYS REVIEWED

Ultraviolet and heat rays have powerful tonic and healing action, which you can enjoy without risk or damage by follow-ing this chapter's advice.

When using natural sunlight as a tonic, expose yourself *gradually*. Use skyshine-bathing as a preliminary. Work up from feet to lower legs to thighs, then to below-the-waist, to entire front surface, and to back, adding a new area of exposure at the end of stepwise movement into the sun each day. Or increase sun exposure to the whole body by two-minute increments. In any case, protect your face from direct sunlight and adjust your sun exposures for time and season. Ignore warmth and instant redness in deciding when you have had enough sun. Use suntan oils as shields, not as potentiators. Protect prominences with yellow petroleum jelly, and take precautions against excess heat.

In wintertime, you can sunbathe effectively by making a plastic protector for a sunny window, skylight or door. The weakness of winter sunlight makes it essential to stick to the midday hours. If you can't manage winter sunbaths, ultraviolet rays may do the trick, especially if you sunbathe mainly for effect on your complexion.

Soothing warmth and tonic action combine to make *homemade body-baker baths* wonderfully refreshing. Ordinary lightbulbs give off heat rays just as penetrating as those from expensive special elements, while a specially-hung blanket traps hot air to form a Turkish bath equivalent. Lightbulb heat alone helps boost circulation and ward off stiffness when used according to certain special techniques. Sexual congestion often yields to a hips-high position with warmth applied to back and legs, which detours blood away from the genital area. A heating pad offers a convenient source of heat rays if you cannot undress, but must be used with considerable caution. Many other "ray" machines do no real good, and you should be cautious about buying or paying to use them.

CHAPTER FOUR

Rejuvenating
Physical Activities

Most North Woods lumberjacks live by the motto: "It's better to *wear* out than to *rust* out."

A lot of them live a long, long time and stay vigorously active until an advanced age. Physical activity tones up your heart and arteries—parts whose sound operation means more to long-lasting vigor than all others combined—and helps keep those organs free of disease. Physical activity strengthens your trunk muscles, from which the worst feelings of fatigue otherwise spring. Physical activity speeds body processes which wash wastes out of worn-out muscles and which rid of your system of weakening poisons. Exhausting, time-consuming or dull calisthenics aren't necessary. Things which you enjoy doing and which fit readily into your schedule can do wonders for your health and vigor.

ACTIVITY AS A HEART AND ARTERY TONIC

When one of your automobile tires goes flat, you cut the casing to ribbons if you run two blocks on it. When you get heart trouble, stressful exertion causes further harm, too. But that doesn't mean that exertion hurts the normal heart, any more than driving your car two blocks ruins its inflated tires. In fact, just the opposite is true: proper exercise helps make your heart and arteries more disease-proof, and even aids your recovery from many kinds of severe attack after the original mending process is complete.

The fear that exertion may push you into a heart attack does tremendous harm. By keeping you less active, it actually predisposes you to the very types of trouble you strive to avoid. It isn't *exertion* which makes heart muscle shrink away. It isn't *exertion* which lets detour passages in your network of arteries slowly close over from years of disuse. It isn't *exertion* which lets blood flow become so sluggish that clots form in important vessels. *Inactivity* causes all of these changes, and proper physical activity can reverse or prevent them.

To quash all vestiges of fear that you might damage your heart by staying active, look at these facts:

When physically active workers like mail carriers or freightyard workers are compared with physically inactive workers with matching status and pay like postal clerks and train announcers, the active workers have less than half as many heart attacks, and also have less trouble getting over the attacks they suffer.

You are much more likely to get a heart attack while sound asleep than during the next eight hours after unusual exertion. Newspaper accounts of men who drop dead while shoveling snow in a blizzard or on the first day of the hunting season take no account of the vast numbers performing such exertions, of whom an equal or larger number would probably have heart attacks if they were sitting home in their living rooms. **Unless you have had definite evidence of heart disease, you can increase the vigor of your physical activities in perfect safety. You can include distinct exertions in your program if you so desire. You will not increase your risk of having a heart attack by so doing.**

How to build up heart health. Whenever your heart pumps a little harder than usual, some of its reserve muscle fibers go into action. Previously unused blood vessels open up. If you use these reserve fibers and vessels regularly every day or two, they soon become a permanent part of your heart's equipment. They remain constantly ready to serve you in case of need.

You can actually *build up your heart's strength and its capacity to resist the commonest type of heart attack* in this way.

Unfortunately, you cannot depend on your everyday work to keep your heart strong. Only your body's biggest muscle masses use enough fuel to spur heart action. Machines and other work-saving devices have made most work in the modern world depend mainly on strong arms and dexterous fingers rather than on straining backs and pumping legs. You need to walk, to climb stairs, to ride a bicycle, to row a boat, to lift weights, or to work your large leg and back muscles as if you were doing these things, in order to use sufficient fuel quickly enough that your heart will extend itself substantially. Most people find one of three methods works best for fitting such heart-building activity into their lives almost every day:

1. Heart-spurring transportation. One of my friends lives three miles from his place of work. Winter and summer, he always drove his automobile through rush-hour traffic, fought the wheel while he maneuvered into a narrow parking stall, and arrived at his office in about twenty minutes. Then his son left for college, leaving behind a fine bicycle. One sunny day, my friend tried pedaling to work—and made it easily in twelve minutes. He's been pedaling ever since, with considerable benefit to both his morale and his health.

Even plain walking may get you where you're going more rapidly and conveniently than you might suppose. Uncle Sam's Post Office has never found a better means of transportation for short hauls, although they've tested a great many machines. If you work or shop or visit within a mile or so of home, you'll be surprised how little time it takes to *walk* instead of *ride*—and how much better you'll feel after a few weeks of making the effort.

Walking up the stairs to your work place also has its adherents, especially among big-city folks. One big advantage: you can build your program slowly, and control it perfectly to avoid fatigue. If you walk home from work, you almost always have to go all the way right from the first day. But if you start the climb toward the sixth floor, you can still take the elevator after two or three flights while you're getting into condition. As your capacity builds up, you can increase your climbing span.

One last suggestion: you can sometimes get the heart-building stimulation you need simply by lumping all the walking and big-muscle activities you usually perform each day into one "workout" instead of spreading them. This will cause some extra fatigue for the first few weeks until your muscles and circulation adjust, but will often meet your fitness needs without a single extra motion. A housewife who ordinarily breaks up her stair-climbing, wet-clothes-hanging and movement-requiring jobs can deliberately tackle them one after the other in a period of half an hour or so, then relax in a hot tub for a few minutes and finish with a cold shower (which is especially stimulating after exercise and heat have brought blood to your skin surfaces). An office worker or supervisor can often get some heart stimulation out of his few walking-type chores if he concentrates them into one or two brief periods when he "makes his rounds" instead of spreading them through the whole day.

2. Heart-spurring hobbies and sports. A lot of people find hobbies or sports disappointing as vigor-boosters.

"Golf just makes me tired," one of my patients told me, for example. And no wonder! He only gets out once a week, and then misses about half the time because of bad weather or business conflicts. His muscles never have a chance to accustom themselves to sports exertion. Instead of building himself up, he merely wears himself out.

You need to exercise several times a week to improve your physical condition. You don't need to exercise very vigorously— certainly not to the point of exhaustion or later stiffness. But you must exercise *regularly,* every week, rain or shine. And that usually means either an indoor hobby, a quick work-out sport, or a series of alternatives from which you choose the most suitable for rigidly-scheduled occasions.

Here in Minnesota, for instance, nobody can do the same sort of outdoor activity all year around. An active person usually chooses at least one sport or hobby for each season. A man might choose trout fishing in springtime, swimming in summer, hunting in fall and skiing in winter. A woman might prefer gardening in spring, bird-watching in summer, and bowling or ice-skating the rest of the year. But even in our snow-encumbered months, nobody's muscles need go to pot from lack of enjoyable sports and hobbies suited to his own capacities and vigor. There's too much variety from which to choose.

3. Activity for the sake of health alone. An active life pattern soon puts deliberate exercise at the bottom of a long, long list: exertion-involving chores, transportation exercise and half a dozen sports must fail to materialize before you take exercise for its own sake. But if your interests and circumstances do not spur you to regular activity, concern for your future health should still drive you toward a few minutes of exercise every day or two. If you find that two days have passed without any fairly vigorous and sustained period of activity, you can choose from among several simple programs. The most readily available, rain or shine, is *stair climbing*—the activity doctors use to test your heart's response to exercise because it always stimulates circulation but can readily be regulated to throw no strain on any reasonably healthy heart. If you haven't been very active in recent years, this provides an easy way to build up slowly. You can climb on a very slow count and stop after a very short time for a few days, then gradually build your exertions to match your improved capacities.

When climbing stairs for heart-strengthening purposes, you should not use an entire flight, since the long uphill climb will make you lose your wind before you have extended yourself very much. Use only the bottom four to six steps of a flight, preferably one with a sturdy banister. Go up slowly and deliberately, then turn and descend at the same rate. Turn and ascend again, counting a slow "one, two, three" cadence. To avoid dizziness, turn one way at the top and the other at the bottom. Set a kitchen timer or watch the clock carefully to govern time—two minutes followed by a rest and then two minutes more makes a good exercise period for people who have been very inactive, while ten minutes steady gives a fair work-out to an athletically inclined man or woman.

Next to stair-climbing, the most readily available heart-strengthener is probably the outdoor hike. If fear of falls keeps you in during winter, a pair of calked boots or walking shoes may be worth while. Warm clothing certainly helps, too, although the fear of catching cold through exposure has no sound basis. People feel chilly just before cold symptoms appear because the disease is already coming on, rather than because chilling causes the disease. A raincoat and galoshes make a sound investment, too. With these simple pieces of equipment, you can probably take a constitutional almost any day of the year without hazard to your health and with considerable enjoyment.

If sore feet or unsuitable surroundings make stair-climbing and outdoor hikes inconvenient, use the home variety rowing machine described later in this chapter (p. 68-71). Adjust the weights so that they draw you toward the wall when you bend your knees. Bend and straighten your legs to get rowing action, keeping your back almost entirely upright. By placing most of the burden upon your legs, you will find that you can row slowly for two minutes or so without later muscle soreness, and work up to about ten minutes per day over a period of a month.

FATIGUE-FIGHTING EXERCISES

Every doctor hears this story several times a week:

"It just seems as if I've lost all my starch. A few minutes on my feet leave me exhausted. I clean my house in fits and starts—one or two rooms and I'm ready to sit down. Don't enjoy shopping anymore—I run out of steam even before I run out of money. And if I do anything at all, my back starts to ache like a sore tooth a little later in the day."

If that sounds like you talking, a few special exercises will probably help you tremendously. Undue fatigue and nagging backache very frequently come from poor tone in the muscles of your trunk. The narrow and floppy spinal column is the only bony link between your rib cage and hips. Only your trunk muscles keep your chest upright and give you a rigid base upon which to move your arms and legs. If your abdominal and back muscles are weak or flabby, a few minutes of special exercise each day usually restores your vigor and comfort inside three or four weeks, besides improving your general health. Before starting these exercises, you should be sure that no real disorder is present—fatigue and backache can also come from anemia, poor nutrition, glandular disorders and a host of other conditions which your doctor can readily correct for you. But if a medical checkup shows nothing organically wrong, you can straighten out the difficulty in a hurry with one of these three programs:*

1. A home-made rowing machine. When the fishing season opens on Minnesota's 14,215 lakes, almost every boat in the state has tenants. Most of the youngsters chase fish in lackadaisical, motorized comfort: but the real old-timers stick to their oars. The unbroken quiet, the slow, soothing rhythm, the feeling of strength and power which comes when you use your body's

---

* The usual back and abdomen exercises may do more harm than good because of two glaring defects: First, many of them—lying on your stomach and raising your head and feet off the floor, for instance—involve increasing the hollow in the lower part of your back, which makes it much more subject to injury. Exercises which help you eliminate this hollow for good, or at least eliminate it while your muscles are being contracted, make backstrain quite unlikely. Second, many trunk exercises involve lifting weights or performing maneuvers which overload the spine's joints. None of the activities recommended here have either of these faults.

largest muscle masses—these are rewards enough for the expenditure of a little energy, as many a grizzled North-woodsman stoutly testifies.

You can't enjoy the refreshing breezes and the slap of gentle waves on a swaying hull within the confines of your home, but you can get the same physical benefits our old oarsmen enjoy. Rowing gives pleasant, soothing and not too strenuous exercise which strengthens exactly the muscles most crucial to physical vigor and youthful appearance. It tones up flabby backs and snugs up sagging tummies. You can enjoy these benefits right in your own home without investing more than a few dollars in equipment, by building a home rowing machine.

A home rowing machine has four main parts: something moveable to sit on, something to push your feet against, something to grip and pull upon, and a way of increasing or decreasing the load. Here's how to provide each of them:

a. A moveable seat. Install a set of swiveled 3 to 4 inch casters, preferably of the type made for a garage creeper (priced at under $3 at mail order houses), on the four corners of the seat from a wooden stool or chair, or on a well-sanded piece of hardwood board about 10 x 8 inches.

b. A footrest. An ordinary wall works fine. If you need a little extra room, lay a small table or bench on its side with its legs set on the wall.

c. Grips and pulleys. Sit on your creeper with your feet against the wall or footrest, and reach forward. Attach a pulley to the wall at the two points where your fingertips touch. Hang two other pulleys from the ceiling above. Thread clothesline rope into each ceiling pulley and down through the arm-level ones. Fit with wooden pull-rope handles (or homemade substitutes).

d. Load. Weights attached to the free end of the two ropes provide the resistance or load against which your muscles work. If you have lead or metal weights available, use them. Window weights or old flatirons work just fine. If you want to make weights inexpensively, tin cans full of cement or plaster work very well. Use large juice-cans from which the tops have been cleanly removed. Twist a piece of clotheshanger wire into a loop with the free ends down in the can. Fill with cement or plaster and let set.

Since most people set up their rowing machine in a basement or garage, the rubbing of weights against the wall usually creates no big problem. If you need to protect the walls, a cage of four or five pieces of baling wire strung from ceiling to floor makes a good track for the rising and falling cement-filled cans. Or you can place your ceiling pulleys out into the room a bit, and off to one side.

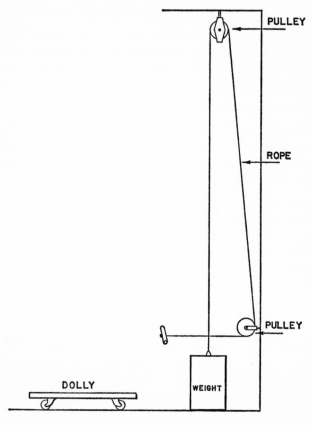

PULLEY

ROPE

PULLEY

DOLLY

WEIGHT

Using your rowing machine. Attach a weight to each rope and sit on your creeper with feet against the wall or footrest. Lean forward and grasp both handles. For the first few sessions, you can keep rowing exercises mild by using fairly heavy weights —heavy enough to counterbalance your upper body when you lean back—and by leaning back only a few degrees on each stroke. Straighten your legs and lean back somewhat—not too far for the first few weeks—pulling the weights up into the air. Let the weights do most of the work in bringing you back to the upright position and in bending your knees to resume starting position, since your abdominal muscles probably will become stiff if you over-use them. A minute or two of slow rowing is quite enough for the first time, and an even slower start is wise if your muscles are quite weak or if you get stiff after trying a minute-long period. Increase very gradually to ten minutes of steady stroking over a period of at least four weeks. If the cord rubs between your fingers to cause soreness or blisters, wear cotton work gloves while rowing.

2. Trunk muscle building sports and hobbies. Your trunk muscles contract when you move any body part against strong resistance, whether you swing a heavy axe or drag your arm through crystal-clear water while swimming. Here's a list of sports and hobbies which definitely build up or maintain the strength of your trunk muscles.

Set-your-own-pace-sports:

Swimming	Croquet
Bowling	Lawn bowling
Golf	Curling
Driving range golf shots	Boccie
Pitch and putt courses	Skiddles (stick bowling)
Rowing	Hiking or walking
Bicycling	Hunting
Skating, ice or roller	Horseback riding
Horseshoe pitching	Quoits
Shuffleboard	

Semi-calisthenic sports:

Card-in-hat game (flip cards into hat, pick up misses one at a time)

Roof-ball game (played with tennis balls and a gentle sloping roof—throw one ball up on roof, then throw another before catching the first and so forth, switching to three balls if you get too good for the two-ball variety)

Hoop rolling (roll a hoop around the house, around the block, or around the neighborhood without letting it fall. Husky men can use an old tire instead of a hoop, with a cotton work glove for hand protection)

Pressure-involving or vigorous sports—good after milder activities have put you into good condition:

Skiing	Softball
Ping-pong	Deck tennis
Badminton	Fencing
Squash	Volleyball
Tennis	Square dancing
Handball	Canoeing

Walk-and-pull-or-stoop hobbies:

Dog-walking	Shell collecting

Bird-watching and other forms of nature study

Rock hounding or agate hunting

One-man's-work, another man's recreation:

Brick laying (like Winston Churchill)

Tree trimming (like Adlai Stevenson)

Wood chopping (a Minnesota favorite)

Upholstering

Furniture refinishing (especially antiques)

Hobbies:

Gardening

Weaving

Rug making (braid-weave or hooked)

Camping

Wood-working

Stone carving

Some kinds of metalwork

3. Push-pull trunk-muscle builders. You can build up your trunk muscles with exercises of a sort well suited to odd moments without wasting any time, although you won't have too much fun in the process. You can fight both weak-tummy-muscle fatigue and lax-muscle paunch with this simple exercise, easily done any time and any place without removing a stitch of clothes:

> Sit upright with both feet flat on the floor. With your arms straight, place both hands, one on top of the other, on your left knee. Press straight down toward the floor without leaning forward. You'll feel your abdominal muscles tighten. Continue smooth, firm pressure for about ten seconds. Relax while switching hands to the right knee. Repeat as on the left. Return to the left, and repeat the whole routine five times.

Back muscles are somewhat harder to exercise without equipment, because they are so strong that you cannot easily counter them with arm pull. About the best anyplace-and-anytime exercise for back muscles goes like this:

> While sitting upright with both feet on the floor, clasp your hands together in front of your right knee. Pull your shoulders up and back, simultaneously pushing down with your thigh muscles to keep your foot on the floor. Continue for ten seconds, then change to the left knee and repeat. Carry out the whole routine three to five times.

You can exercise back muscles more effectively if odd moments find you alone in your house, office or shop. With privacy and a wall to lean against, this simple exercise lets body weight rather than arm pull resist your back muscles' contraction:

> Leaning your back against a wall, edge your feet forward until they are about eighteen inches from the baseboard. Roll your hips forward in a sort of burlesque

bump while simultaneously stretching the back of the top
of your head toward the ceiling—this flattens the back
against the wall in its strongest position. Place both
hands on your hips. Without changing trunk alignment,
bring your hips forward until your back is straight, your
body extended on a diagonal from your feet to your upper back. Move your hips very slowly in an eight-inch
circle, being careful not to carry them so far forward
that a hollow forms in your low back—if your hips roll
forward or back in their alignment with your body, lean
back against the wall to align your spinal column properly once more. Rotate your hips ten times in this position, then turn so that your right shoulder rather than
your upper back rests against the wall, with your feet
(now parallel to the wall) still eighteen inches away from
the mopboard. Slowly rotate your hips through an eight-
inch circle for ten more revolutions. Turn the left shoulder toward the wall and do the same. This exercise may
be made somewhat more strenuous by moving the feet
farther from the wall, or somewhat milder by keeping
them closer. The hands-on-hips posture is important,
because it makes you aware of any change in back and
hip alignment.

Repeat the routine three times on the first go-round,
and wait a day or so to see if any stiffness results before
trying again. Build up to five repetitions of the procedure,
performing it very slowly and deliberately.

Strong trunk muscles ward off fatigue and backache so effectively that most people find the time spent on daily exercises
more than worthwhile. A few weeks of daily trunk-muscle activity will almost certainly leave you feeling fresh and vigorous
all through the day and evening—a real difference from the logy,
worn-out feeling which so many people blame on inevitable
middle age.

HOW TO DRAIN AWAY FATIGUE AND DISCOMFORT

When a muscle gets weary, acid wastes pile up inside each microscopic fibril. These wastes lead to weakness and fatigue: when you flush them out, you make the muscle strong and comfortable again. That's why exercises which drain away acid wastes relieve exhaustion almost instantaneously, unlike exercises that depend on improved condition and increased strength.

Perhaps the most useful such exercise aids leg-weariness, particularly after prolonged standing or walking. Stagnation in the veins adds to the waste accumulation. A thorough vein-flush helps a lot.

> Take off your shoes and socks. Lie on your back with your hips propped up either on the arm of a davenport or on your hands (with your elbows braced on the floor). Stretch your legs straight toward the ceiling and let the muscles of your feet and ankles go completely loose. Jiggle the feet in rapid vibrating motions, imparting motion with the muscles of the thigh rather than those controlling the foot and ankle itself (which should remain ragdoll loose and floppy). After fifteen seconds, stop this motion and encircle your right ankle with the thumbs and forefingers of your two hands. Slide your hands up along your leg to your knee, pressing gently into the flesh to milk body fluids along their way toward the body. Repeat three times, then do the same with the left leg. Jiggle the feet for fifteen seconds longer, then resume your clothing and go on your way. You'll find your legs greatly refreshed.

Breathing exercises work similarly to blow off fatigue-causing waste products accumulated in your blood. They help most for brain-work fatigue—the weariness that overtakes you after wrestling with your income tax forms or writing an important letter. The lack of physical exertion during brainwork tends to make your breathing shallow, and shallow breathing gives gaseous wastes little chance to escape through your lungs. These gaseous wastes make you feel dull, logy and fatigued, as if you have cobwebs in the brain. Eight or ten deep breaths often give relief. Stand with one hand on your abdomen and the other on your hip. Take in air through your nose, first by contracting the diaphragm, which pushes your organs downward and makes your abdomen more prominent. Finish the intake of air by expanding your chest to its limit. Let the air out unforced through your mouth, and repeat for a total of ten breaths. If you feel dizzy or light-headed, you have breathed too fast. The sensation will pass quickly, and can be avoided on future occasions by going more slowly.

EXERCISE AND ELIMINATION

Although you cannot improve elimination of sluggishly moving bowel contents within minutes like accumulated muscle and blood-borne gaseous wastes, physical activity encourages normal bowel action over a period of time. Two factors seem important: the gentle massage of abdominal contents which comes from contraction of the muscles in the vicinity, and improved muscle tone which gives your inner organs better support. For the first purpose, ordinary walking does as well as anything: alternate contraction of muscles in front of the backbone on the two sides massages the last few segments of bowel much more effectively than any external friction. A twenty-minute walk each day plus the dietary and bulk-producing measures discussed in Chapters Six and Seven add up to an excellent, completely natural means of bowel regulation. The trunk exercises described earlier in this chapter improve abdominal muscle tone, which also helps to combat sluggish bowel.

CHAPTER FOUR'S MAIN POINTS ABOUT
REJUVENATING ACTIVITY

Physical activity helps you toward:

1. A longer-lasting heart. Exertion doesn't hurt a normal heart at any age. Mild exertions help to build up and maintain heart strength, open detour passages to prevent the coronary artery blockage which causes most heart attacks. Bicycling, walking, and lumped exercise-involving chores often fit readily into your daily schedule. Hobbies and sports often help, too, especially if you include choices for each season and both indoor and outdoor varieties. When these do not suffice, fulfill your need for heart-building exercise with stair-climbing, hiking or indoor rowing.

2. Greater vigor and endurance. Trunk muscle strength and tone has a great deal to do with fatigue. You'll probably gain extra energy and vigor from activities which strengthen your back and abdomen, such as rowing on a home-made machine, trunk-muscle-building sports and hobbies, and push-pull trunk-muscle builders.

3. Flush away fatigue and misery. Drain away acid wastes from weary leg muscles with the limp-foot-shaking exercise. Air-wash your lungs free of products of brain-work stagnation and fatigue. Use mild, daily exercise such as walking to control constipation, along with measures suggested in Chapters Six, Seven and Eight.

CHAPTER FIVE

New Vigor and
Tranquility Through
Muscular Control

People who continually worry generally know that the energy they spend on fretting and stewing would go a long way toward solving their problems. A harried housewife racing from stove to telephone to misbehaving child knows that haste and pressure exhaust her more than housework itself. Even the worn-out laborer may realize that the tension of wondering how he can meet next month's car and furniture payments sometimes exhausts him more than eight hours on the job.

Each of these people sadly says:

"I know I'm racing my motor psychologically. But I don't know how to quit. You can't tell yourself 'Keep calm!' Human nature doesn't work that way."

One hundred per cent correct! Your intellect can't turn emotions on and off at will. But almost all strength- and efficiency-sapping emotions share one major ingredient which you *can* turn off at will. *Muscular tension* is an integral part of these emotions, through which they do most of their harm and without which they often quickly fade. And muscular tension is very much subject to deliberate control.

MUSCULAR RELAXATION

Your brain commands muscles to contract and to relax hundreds of times each hour. It can use this power at any time, even when emotions have previously held command. And muscular response is so much a part of an emotion that lessening muscular tension often soothes the feelings which originally created it. That's one of the great secrets of the Indian mystics whose ability to go without sleep and endure discomfort is almost legendary: they soothe the mind by relaxing their bodies instead of combatting nervous pressures and upheavals by futile attempts at direct self-mastery.

Gain energy, comfort, cheerfulness and resiliency through relaxation. If you feel tired by the end of the day, chances are that tension is partially at fault. Tense muscles use as much energy as overworked ones. In fact, moderate tension makes sitting in a chair as much work as walking steadily uphill when thoroughly relaxed.

If you get headaches, nagging backache, or migrating aches and pains, tension may well be at fault. Muscles become stiff from tension as quickly as from exercise. Your scalp and back muscles are especially likely to show effects, causing considerable discomfort.

Even if tension does not cause fatigue or muscle pain, it makes you miserable. Keyed up, nervous feelings usually disappear with muscular relaxation, even though the circumstances which set them off remain unchanged. And if nervousness has kept you from working out your problems, the tranquility you gain through relaxation may provide you a firm base from which to operate.

Relaxation costs you nothing. Perhaps tension served a useful function in centuries past. When a caveman had reason to be anxious, he needed every muscle on alert: the extra tautness of muscular tension made him ready for quick action without a lag for taking up muscular slack. However, lightning-fast action often does more harm than good nowadays. It's better to think before you leap in this modern age. Leap-before-you-look reflexes won't get you out of trouble very often, and thought-impairing nervous tension will often get you into it.

Even when you feel no notable tension and are making no deliberate use of a body part, its muscles keep themselves somewhat taut. Relaxing this residual tautness helps increase your energy and make you proof against upset. Relaxation restores your vigor three to four times as fast as ordinary napping and clears the cobwebs out of your brain instead of leaving you feeling in a fog. In terms of time, deliberate relaxation costs you almost nothing. You can do a lot of relaxing in odd moments which would otherwise go to waste. And decreased need for sleep more than repays you for the useful time you spend on relaxation.

Learning to relax. The actual technique for relaxing seems easiest to learn in the range of muscular contraction with which everyone is familiar—that of deliberate stiffness or muscle use. Once you know how to relax a muscle in this range, you can easily apply the lesson to rid yourself of unintentional muscle tautness or tension. Here's a good starting procedure:

> While lying flat on a comfortable bed or davenport, hold your neck a little bit stiff, somewhat stiffer yet, and then as stiff as you can manage. Relax again in stages to somewhat stiff, a little bit stiff, and your usual level of tautness, *then carry the same process one step further, loosening the muscle beyond its normal state of expectant tautness.* Do this several times, until you get the "feel" of relaxation.

TECHNIQUES OF RELAXATION

If you've ever tried to relax your whole body at once, you know that it is almost impossible. The extra burden of attempted self-control only increases tension, and annoyance at your inevitable failure adds further misery.

You *can* relax. But you must bring your mental energies to bear on only one part of your body at a time in order to relax it.

Relax part-by-part. All successful ways of relaxing share one characteristic: they concentrate on one body part at a time. You can do this quite easily by following a simple system: relax each extremity in around-the-clock order, then relax your head and trunk from top to bottom. In succession, relax your right arm, right leg, left leg, left arm, scalp, forehead, face, neck, chest, back and abdomen.

Relax step-by-step. A single, casual self-command dissipates a certain portion of the tension in any muscle, but seldom brings it from a state of annoying overtautness to complete relaxation. You cannot make further progress by trying harder: straining (even toward relaxation) defeats the purpose. But you *can* achieve further relaxation by making several distinct and separate efforts. The first of these efforts will reduce muscle tautness to some degree. The next will pick up where the first left off and achieve a further degree of relaxation. After several distinct efforts, your muscles will be much more thoroughly relaxed than would otherwise have been possible.

Fortunately, you can achieve several successive degrees of relaxation quite easily by concentrating in rotation on one body part or area at a time. By the time you have finished an around-the-clock-and-top-to-bottom routine, you'll find that a fresh start picks up where the first round left off and partially relieves the remaining muscle tautness. A second round carries relaxation one step further, and so on.

The invigorating interval. You can reap benefits from deliberate relaxation most easily during an "invigorating interval." Choose a time when tension has already piled up to some degree—the lunch or before-supper hour if you have a regular job, perhaps the lag which precedes the supper-preparation rush if you're a housewife. Take off your shoes and loosen your clothing to make yourself entirely comfortable. Lie down in a quiet, darkened room. Practice the art of relaxing with the stiff-neck method described above (p. 82) unless you have already thoroughly mastered it, then focus your mental energies on relaxing one body part after another in around-the-clock, top-to-bottom order. Relax your right arm, right leg, left leg, left arm, scalp, forehead, face, neck, chest, back and abdomen until you have eased tautness in every muscle in your body. Immediately begin another round, striving for even further relaxation. You might set an alarm clock so that you don't have to keep track of time, but you'll probably find it unnecessary: most people don't really go to sleep in this type of relaxation interval, hanging in a state of tranquil semi-consciousness in which they are not particularly aware of the passage of time but still become alert almost instantly when the allotted number of minutes has passed. Relax for about twenty minutes at a time. When you get up and go about your business, you'll feel greatly refreshed and invigorated—much more so than after an actual nap. If you find yourself feeling dopey or fuzzy-headed after relaxation, shorten your invigorating interval to fifteen minutes, or even to ten. A brisk cold-water face bath helps to restore clear-headedness while you're feeling for the interval that best suits your own needs.

When you feel quite keyed up or have been under unusual pressure, you may find it hard to relax completely. Under such circumstances, simply focus your mental energies on smaller portions of your body at a time. Instead of trying to relax your right arm as a unit, relax your right hand, then your wrist, then your forearm, then your upper arm, and then your shoulder. You'll find that even high grades of emotional turmoil and anxiety yield to this technique.

Breathing and relaxation. Readily-mastered breathing exercises often help to ease tension and limit its harmful after-effects. Some of the most troublesome results of tension come from tautness in the breathing muscles. Tightness in the chest and a feeling of smothering oppression often plague you during moments of high tension. Aches and pains in the chest follow periods of stress and strain, mainly because prolonged tautness in the breathing muscles makes them stiff from overwork. Fuzzy-headedness and loss of appetite sometimes result when gaseous wastes pile up in the bloodstream due to shallow, tension-limited respiration, which also presses you toward excessive smoking—

tobacco smoke increases depth and speed of respiration by irritating nerve endings in your lungs, thus indirectly (and often at high price in health) giving some of the same benefits as breathing exercises. Excessive breathing-muscle tautness also causes backache, stiff neck, and general exhaustion by throwing muscle pull out of balance and increasing strain.

You put a stop to all this when you breathe deeply and regularly for half a minute or more. Simply stand erect near a window with your right hand on your abdomen and your left hand on your hip. Breathe in through your nose, at first leaving the chest muscles completely relaxed and inflating your lungs with your diaphragm, the muscular sheet dividing chest from tummy. You'll feel the abdomen bulge forward as the diaphragm draws itself downward. When you have filled your lungs as far as possible by this maneuver, slowly expand your chest like a bellows. When you cannot draw in another sniff of air, let your lungs empty themselves through your partially opened mouth. Do not forcibly exhale: simply let the air escape from your chest's unaided elasticity. Repeat ten to twelve times, either as a relaxing general refresher or as a follow-up to an "invigorating interval."

The refresher slouch. After you have practiced the art of relaxing during "invigorating intervals" and learned to ease breathing-muscle tension with special exercises, you can put these two skills together in a quick and easy technique which breaks the build-up of tension and restores considerable energy. The "refresher slouch" takes two minutes or less, and can be done right at your desk or in any comfortable chair. While a single "slouch" doesn't match the effect of an "invigorating interval," ten to twenty minutes in short breaks probably do you at least as much good as the same time spent all at once in bed-bound relaxation. And two-minute refreshers fit into odd moments when you wouldn't accomplish anything anyway, like subway station waits, the tag end of the lunch hour, and uninteresting TV commercials. The details:

Sit with both feet flat on the ground and both hands resting on top of your thighs. Let your head loll forward and your eyes fall shut. Relax your right arm, right leg and so on in around-the-clock-then-top-to-bottom order. Take a deep breath through your nose, drawing down your diaphragm without expanding your chest to get as much air into your lungs as possible, then inflating still further by chest expansion. Let the air escape unforced through your mouth, and begin another round of body relaxation. Continue in this fashion for about two minutes, or until you feel fully relaxed and rested.

Yoga exercises. As part of a system of self-mastery, yoga has much different aims than body-building or fitness-promoting exercises. Since everyone can govern muscle *contractions* fairly well, it tries to improve control by emphasizing muscle *relaxation*. After centuries of trial and error, the Eastern mystics have found certain exercises best for leaving the troubles and worries of the world behind them, for enlivening the mind and for revitalizing the body. While you cannot accomplish the whole yoga routine without months of gradual stretching, anyone can do several key exercises which offer rich rewards in emotional tranquility, mental enlivenment and physical invigoration.

1. The back-stretching leg pull. Sit on the floor with your legs straight and your feet together. Bend your trunk slowly forward, then grasp your legs with both hands as far down as you can reach. Bend your head forward. Pull slowly and gently with both arms as if trying to draw the top of your head toward your feet. Stretch as far as you can without discomfort, and hold this position for a count of five seconds. You'll find muscles easier to stretch if you concentrate on relaxing your back and neck rather than on pulling with your arms. Don't worry if you can't pull yourself down into a closed-jack-knife position at first: this exercise helps a lot even if you barely reach your knees. After five seconds, sit up and take one or two deep breaths, then repeat the exercise. A total of three stretches makes a full and adequate set.

2. *The thigh stretch.* Sit on an inch-thick kneeling pad or cushion. Use a folded towel if no pad is available. Place the soles of your feet flat against each other, bending your knees to draw your heels up close to your crotch. Fold your hands together, then clasp them around your arches. Sitting quite upright, pull straight upward with your hands, simultaneously spreading and depressing your thighs. Maintain the push-pull pressure for a count of five seconds, then allow your legs to relax. Repeat three times.

3. *The tension-easing grimace.* Deliberate face-muscle contraction and relaxation helps to soothe tension, diminish wrinkle-causing facial sag, and combat high-pressure-living headaches. The tension-easing grimace quickly relieves taut scalp and face muscles, and simultaneously builds up their strength so that the overload of future tension will not make them sore. Since scalp muscle stiffness causes most tension-type headache, this greatly aids your future comfort. Improved muscle tone also gives more youthful appearance.

While comfortably seated, lean slightly forward. Open your eyes as wide as possible. Draw your eyebrows and your ears upward toward the top of your head. Open your mouth wide, pulling its corners toward your ears. Protrude your tongue hard, with its tip pointed toward your chin. Throw your shoulders back and stiffen your chest. Spread your fingers as wide as possible. Hold this position for a count of five full seconds, with muscles of the eyelids, scalp, face, tongue and hands as stiff as possible. Slump into the "refresher slouch" position described above, with eyes closed, head lolling forward and hands resting on your thighs, for five seconds, relaxing thoroughly. Alternate the grimace with the slouch for five repetitions. After a few weeks of practice, you can build the duration of the grimace phase to fifteen or twenty seconds on each repetition if a tendency toward facial sag or headache makes the extra effort seem worthwhile.

4. *Nostril-controlled respiration.* Centuries before modern sci-

ence "discovered" certain reflexes, yoga used them for tonic and tranquilizing effects. Nostril-controlled respiration is an excellent example: by gently increasing the suction within the chest during inspiration and the pressure within the chest during the breath-holding and expiration phase, it massages the great veins and auricles. Half a dozen Western scientists have attached their names to the bodily mechanisms involved, but none has found a better way to improve the brain's circulation, banish the muddle-headedness of first awakening, soothe jangled nerves and simultaneously enliven mind and spirit.

Place the first and second fingers of one hand on the bridge of your nose. The thumb and other two fingers will rest against the sides of your nose in such a way that slight pressure will close off either nostril. Close off the left nostril and slowly but steadily draw in a deep breath. First fill the lungs as far as possible with the diaphragm, which moves downward and makes the abdomen bulge while the rib cage remains stationary. Then expand the chest itself to draw in a complete breath. This should be done slowly, taking six to ten seconds. When your lungs have filled to capacity, close off both nostrils. Retain the air for six to ten seconds, not by holding the chest muscles and diaphragm tense but by keeping all outlets through the nose and mouth entirely closed. Relax your breathing muscles as completely as possible during this phase, letting the chest's elastic recoil create gentle pressure on the retained air and thus on the great veins within the chest. This milks half-stagnant blood into the heart and improves the circulation. Now release the right nostril and let the air gently escape, trying to make the exhalation last another six to ten seconds. Repeat, inhaling this time through the just-used right nostril and exhaling through the left. Perform the whole cycle seven times, for a total of fourteen breaths. If you find yourself becoming giddy or light-headed, make each breathing phase longer—say fifteen seconds—to prevent overventilation.

5. Advanced yoga. If exercises 1-4 give you distinct benefits, you may want to carry on to more difficult and time-consuming routines. Yoga includes over two dozen push-pull or balance-against-gravity-and-muscle-strain postures, besides countless breathing exercises and mental or philosophical drills. Supple Orientals cross their legs with both ankles resting on the fronts of their thighs. Veteran practitioners stand upside down, resting on head or shoulders, for half an hour at a time. These and other exercises have definite relaxing, invigorating, and circulation-aiding value. Since you need daily practice for weeks or months to accomplish them, however, specific directions seem best left for manuals devoted entirely to the subject.

Continual relaxation. After a good deal of practice with various methods of relaxation, you will find that you can apply some tension-relieving techniques as you go about your usual activities. Since your full mental energies do not apply themselves to any muscle group or part, this method is far more difficult than any of the others. However, the extra vigor and tranquility which it creates make its mastery worthwhile. Real experts can cut their sleep requirement in half, gaining hours of useful endeavor every day, and still feel rested and energetic. Almost everyone can reach a degree of relaxation skill which increases vigor, soothes jumpy nerves and decreases irritability.

How many of your muscle fibers are taut right now, as you sit and read this book? Certainly, a great many more than would be needed to keep your body erect and turn the pages. After a few weeks of "invigorating intervals" and "refresher slouches," you will find yourself able to command unneeded muscles to greater laxity in a mere moment. As you sit at your desk, ride in your car or pull up your chair at the dining room table, you can greatly reduce muscle tautness. A few more weeks of repeated relaxation can make lowered tensions into a habit. Such an effort can often break the tension-begets-more-tension cycle which keeps most modern men and women keyed up to a point of uncomfortable inefficiency. It can change your whole life for the better without consuming a single extra minute of time, once proper patterns have become ingrained.

CHAPTER FIVE'S MAIN POINTS ABOUT MUSCULAR CONTROL

You can't control emotion directly through exercise of intellect or will, but you can indirectly soothe most tension and anxiety by controlling its muscular elements. In the process, you'll gain strength and energy, avoid nagging discomforts, and think out problems more clearly. All at no real cost in efficiency or time.

Learn the art of relaxation first by moving between degrees of deliberate stiffness. Focus your attention on one muscle group at a time while trying to relax. Follow around-the-clock and top-to-bottom order, relaxing one body part at a time. Apply this technique during "invigorating intervals"—periods set apart, when you get away from all distractions and discomforts to make relaxation easier. Follow your "invigorating interval" with breathing exercises—a complete abdomen-first-and-chest-afterwards breath about ten times running. Use breathing exercises by themselves for a quick refresher and tension easer—they're available any place and at any time. So is the "refresher slouch," a chairbound combination of relaxation and breathing exercises which you can manage in two minutes flat once you have mastered the basic techniques.

Yoga exercises also help you to relax, clear your mind and gain vigor. You can easily learn the back-stretching leg pull, the thigh stretch, the tension-easing grimace and nostril-controlled respiration. More advanced exercises are available if you want to pursue the subject.

After grounding yourself thoroughly in specific relaxation techniques, you will probably find that you can control the build-up of tension to some extent as you go along, without taking time out for specific procedures. Both the special relaxation techniques and the aid they give you in minute-by-minute self-control add greatly to your mental and physical comfort, your capability and your vigor.

CHAPTER SIX

Natural Foods for
Health and Vigor

1. Depend on natural food, not pills and potions 94, 2. Count food groups, not fuel values 95, 3. Count 4-5-5 for greater vigor 96, 4. Eat often for energy 99, 5. Use your quick-energy snacks to fill your food count 99, 6. Boost reserve-energy foods 100, 7. Replace table spreads, shortening and fats or oils with quicker energy foods whenever possible 101, 8. Dodge chemically treated fats for long-term tonic action 102, 9. Eat foods in a form you can readily chew 103, 10. Regulate your bowels the natural way 103, Summary 105.

If you turn into a Minnesota farmer's driveway, the scrunch of gravel beneath your tires triggers a burst of activity. Before she even knows who is coming, the housewife plucks the bubbling kettle from the corncob-fired cookstove and fills the reservoir of a drip coffee pot. Layer cake or fresh rolls appear on the big kitchen table, and menfolk cluster around it for a friendly exercise of the coffee-drinker's elbow.

The fun of coffee breaks comes from friendly people, but the invigoration comes mainly from food. Hard-working farmers don't begrudge snack time, even if it means plowing with headlights far into the night. The quick lift, the surge of strength, the fresh energy make any excuse good enough to justify an extra feed. You can certainly perk yourself up with energy-yielding fuels even when no social occasion inspires you. Both at mealtimes and between, the greatest tonics come from the grocery rather than the drugstore, and you only need ten simple rules to make the most of them.

I. DEPEND ON NATURAL FOOD, NOT PILLS AND POTIONS

No chemist alive can manufacture many of the most important substances which your body needs. At least a few important elements probably remain entirely unidentified: nutritionists do not even claim the power to mix a sludge of manufactured chemicals upon which an animal or man can thrive as well as upon natural foods. A natural food program can do more for you than *any* artificial food supplement, no matter what its price. And in cost, of course, there's no comparison.

94

2. COUNT FOOD GROUPS, NOT FUEL VALUES

When you think about food as fuel, the family automobile seems an apt comparison. A car runs as long as there's gas in the tank, and you don't need to put in portions of twenty different brands to keep it going. But the human body works more like a complicated factory than like a single motor. It needs power-giving fuel for all its machinery, but it also needs special supplies for a hundred different assembly lines. Even a single missing item throws the whole operation out of kilter. Maybe you can turn out the needed part in another division, or redesign the product. But you can't operate as effectively as you could if all your needs were met.

Varied food is a time-bomb tonic. Frequent servings from each important natural food group can make you feel better and accomplish more within a week or two, even although you don't see an immediate effect. And you don't need weird foods or chemicals: systematic use of items which every grocer carries will fill the bill.

Use your five fingers to help remember which foods you need each day. Meat, vegetables, fruit, dairy products and foods made from grain each provide different body-needed supplies. Learn to tick these five groups off on your fingers, and a tonic-food program for greater strength and vigor becomes quite easy. Meat, vegetables, fruit, dairy products and grain. Servings of each in rotation means much-improved vigor and health.

3. COUNT 4-5-5 FOR GREATER VIGOR

For total time-bomb tonic action, your meals and snacks should provide nearly three servings in each food group every day. You can reach that goal by counting off food groups on your fingers as you go along, without ever keeping records or writing out menus as old-fashioned nutritionists demand.

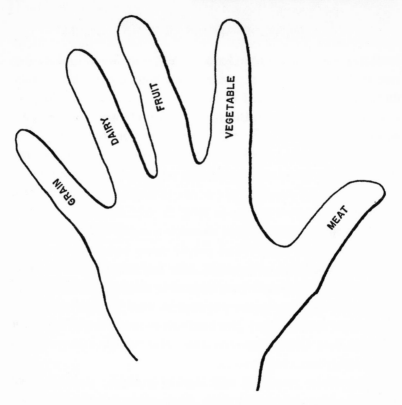

Meat, vegetables, fruit, dairy products and grain.

Start again at the beginning of each meal, and don't count duplications. If you have cereal and milk for breakfast, for instance, you can raise your count by including fruit in a midmorning snack, but not by including milk, which only duplicates a need you have already met.

Count each major ingredient in a combination dish, if the amount is substantial. Beef stew might contain meat, vegetables and potatoes, for instance. A dessert of mandarin oranges, coconut and sour cream scores as both fruit and dairy products because a substantial amount of both are ingredients, but a mere dab of whipped cream on top of a fruit tart does not deserve to be counted. The amount of grain-derived flour used to thicken gravy doesn't score, but the crust on a meat or fruit pie deserves to be counted. Generally speaking, if an ingredient amounts to several spoon- or forkfuls in each serving, it deserves to be scored just as if it were served separate, while amounts much less than this can be neglected.

As to individual food groups, here are answers to the questions which often arise:

Meat: Score eggs, fish and other protein-rich meat substitutes as meat. Even protein-rich vegetable products like peanut butter and seed-type (kidney or red) beans or black-eyed peas can be counted in the meat group as long as you don't use them to replace meat more than once or twice a week.

Vegetables and fruit: Most people score raw tomatoes as a fruit, cooked ones as a vegetable. One leaf of lettuce in a sandwich doesn't really meet your vegetable needs, and should not be counted. I always count potatoes in with "grain" instead of "vegetables" because they give food values much more like those of bread than those of greens (and also because the two are more readily interchangeable).

Dairy: Since you need milk for its proteins, vitamins and minerals rather than its butterfat, don't count butter as a dairy product. Ice cream, cottage cheese and other milk products have less varied food value than whole milk, but meet your needs reasonably well.

Grain: Products made from whole grain, such as whole wheat or cracked wheat bread, rye bread, oatmeal and breakfast cereals, contain up to ten times as much mineral and vitamin as products made from highly refined grain, such as white bread and polished rice. Count any baked product or flour-base food, but try to make as much of it whole-grain as possible.

Let's count out a few meals to make the process clear. The lefthand column shows items you might eat in two successive days. The righthand columns show their food group and a running count.

FOOD	GROUP	COUNT
Breakfast		
Tomato juice	Fruit	1
Eggs	Meat	2
Bacon	Meat	Still 2, since you can't count any group but once for same meal.
Coffee, black	—	—
Toast with butter	Grain	3

(Start over at each meal.)

Lunch		
Ham sandwich	Meat and grain	2
Lettuce salad	Vegetable	3
Milk	Dairy	4
Canned Peaches	Fruit	5
Dinner		
Steak	Meat	1
Potatoes	Grain	2
Green beans	Vegetable	3
Coffee	—	—
Ice Cream	Dairy	4
Breakfast		
Cereal with milk and fruit	Grain, dairy & fruit	3
Coffee	—	—
Lunch		
Cold cuts	Meat	1
Potato salad (with lettuce & celery)	Grain & vegetable	3
Milk	Dairy	4
Apple	Fruit	5
Dinner		
Lamb stew with potato & carrots	Meat, grain, vegetable	3
Cake	Grain (repeater)	—
Coffee	—	—

Against the ideal for full tonic effect of 4-5-5 (four food groups in breakfast, all five in both lunch and supper), these meals fall definitely short. The first day's menus score 3-5-4, the second's 3-5-3. The food group count points out exactly what foods would give further effect on improving your health and energy while you still have time to do something about it, either at meals or through appropriate choice of snacks (see point 5 below). But this system doesn't force you to plan your day's meals a week ahead.

4. EAT OFTEN FOR ENERGY

Take a tip from our midwestern farmers, some of the hardest workers in the world: a midmorning snack can make you feel better and accomplish more right up to lunchtime. By actual measurement, you'll achieve one-tenth more than non-snackers in the last hour of the morning, and a full quarter more than complete non-breakfasters. Between-meals eating can improve both your mental outlook and your physical capacities without adding to your waistline, too. Small amounts of quick-energy food give you a boost and actually soothe your hunger in advance of the next meal.

5. USE YOUR QUICK-ENERGY SNACKS TO FILL YOUR FOOD COUNT

If you have youngsters, you've probably worried about whether snacks might do them harm by cutting out their appetite for more wholesome mealtime dishes. With the kind of snacks most youngsters choose—candy, pop and gum—that's a sound line of thought. Adults can fall into the same pitfall themselves, replacing long-range bracer foods like vegetables and fruits with less helpful cake and rolls. But you don't have to make this mistake. You can use snacks to achieve lasting and impressive invigoration. That's where the 4-5-5 system does its best work—in helping you to choose snacks to give both instant energy and long-range tonic aid.

Suppose, for instance, that you breakfast on eggs and toast (with food-groups "meat" and "grain," totaling 2). A piece of fruit, some ice cream or cheese, or a dish of vegetable soup would increase your morning count from 2 to 3. If you breakfast on cereal, fruit and milk or cream (grain, fruit and dairy), a scoop of chicken salad (meat and vegetable) would boost your count from 3 to 5. You would get all the quick-energy help which rolls and coffee could yield, plus the tonic values of vitamins, proteins and minerals which only a full variety of natural foods can provide.

To tickle your imagination, here are a few lasting-energy snacks which you could easily prepare or carry:

> Sardines, pickled herring, smoked oysters, lunch meat rolled around pickle or olives, small squares of Edam, Swiss or Provolone cheese on toothpicks, ham, shrimp or chicken salad (made with celery and reduction-type whipped dressing if you're watching your weight), vegetable or tossed salad, soup, stew, canned, dried or fresh fruit, ice cream, milk, and cottage cheese either alone or in combination with tomatoes or fruit.

In my own home, we make up a few favorite snack foods in quantity and keep them in the refrigerator or divide them into small portions for freezing. Many of these foods also come in small-sized cans, individual pieces, or shelf-stored and not too spoilable form.

6. BOOST RESERVE-ENERGY FOODS

Look on any menu: the feature dish is meat, fish, cheese or eggs. Protein foods stick to your ribs, not only as body builders and in self-replacement or repair, but as energy reserves. Your body slowly changes most protein into energy-yielding carbohy-drate over a period of several hours. A constant flow of quick-energy fuel enlivens your brain and muscles for a long time after a high protein meal, helping you to stay mentally and physically active without becoming muddle-headed and weary.

The count 4-5-5 system guarantees two or three protein foods every day, since the "meat" group always yields lots of protein. But you can gain still further energy and lasting zoom by working extra protein foods into each meal. Hard boiled and sieve eggs to sprinkle into salads and over vegetables—you'll find a great many dishes made tastier and more satisfying in this way. Mix yogurt with strawberries or other fruits, then freeze in your refrigerator trays for a high-protein snack or dessert. Boost your use of low-cost vegetable proteins by making bean soup and other legume-featuring dishes. Spread sandwiches with a thick layer of cottage cheese instead of using butter. Work protein-containing ingredi-ents like eggs and meat into all your favorite dishes for extra pep and energy.

7. REPLACE TABLE SPREADS, SHORTENING AND FATS OR OILS WITH QUICKER ENERGY FOODS WHENEVER POSSIBLE

As a Minnesotan, I'm supposed to plump for butter. It's one of this state's main products, and a delicious one at that. But as a doctor, I have to do what's best for *you* instead of boosting the state's economy. On these terms, butter deserves only a small chink in your refrigerator. It's true that butter or oleomargarine supplies needed vitamin D for growing bones, but unless you deliberately replace butter and oleomargarine with vitaminless oil in every recipe, you almost can't avoid meeting these needs.

On the other hand, adults need food-boosted energy, while children and adolescents have intrinsic zoom. So it makes sense to replace the thickly buttered bread of a juvenile's sandwich with a quarter-inch layer of cottage cheese, to replace the fried hamburger so dear to youth with a thicker patty of broiled lean meat, and to replace thick-crusted (and shortening-rich) pie with three times as much fresh or canned fruit. Even your steaks and chops can be at least twice as thick without any risk to your figure if you trim off all visible fat.

These changes trade gobs of non-invigorating fat either for reserve-energy-boosting protein or for foods readily used as pick-me-ups all through the day. Suit your own tastes, of course, but make as many protein-and-carbohydrate-for-fat substitutions as you can.

8. DODGE CHEMICALLY TREATED FATS FOR LONG-TERM TONIC ACTION

One of the slyest intrusions of chemical alteration into the food industry occurred with the manufacture of artificially solidified shortenings. Housewives took poorly to vegetable oils at first, so the manufacturers put their safe, natural and healthful product through a chemical process. This process converted liquid oil to solid shortening by changing artery-sustaining *unsaturated* fats into *saturated* fats, which mountains of research now link with hardening of the arteries, coronary heart attacks, stroke and many other ravages formerly blamed upon old age.

The same research which has made a strong case for natural, unaltered vegetable oils has also pointed to other ways of dodging the ravages of hard arteries (which include most of the miseries people have always blamed on "old age"). You can probably enjoy substantial long-range tonic effect—better health for many years when old age approaches—by following three simple rules:

1. Eat *natural* oils and oil-containing products rather than hydrogenated ones whenever possible. This means corn, cotton-seed or sunflower seed oil rather than white manufactured short-

enings, and old fashioned peanut butter instead of "creamy" or "no oil separation" types. You can get the preferred varieties in any good grocery without paying a fancy drugstore price.

2. Trim off visible fat from meats—eat lean part only.

3. Choose low-saturated-fat fish or poultry as your main dish at least twice a week.

You can probably bring your saturated fat intake down to match what people ate before the shortening salesman's chemists went wild, by taking these three simple steps. Ten or twenty years from now, you'll feel the difference in retained vigor and health.

9. EAT FOODS IN A FORM YOU CAN READILY CHEW

You only benefit from food your body digests. Solid chunks of food contribute nothing, and may cause gas pains or other discomforts. Starches also need extra chewing, but for a different reason—your body breaks down starch into digestible sugars only through the action of saliva. So baked goods and potatoes call for slow savoring, not fast demolishment.

A great many of my older patients don't get as much strength and vigor from their food as they really should. Sometimes they find help in medicinal tonics like Taka-Diastase, which digests unchewed starches for them: sometimes they suffer along, feeling and acting older than their years. In either case, the simple habit of thorough chewing, combined with attractive, leisurely meals to aid the flow of saliva and digestive juices, usually ends the problem.

10. REGULATE YOUR BOWELS THE NATURAL WAY

A famous general's one instruction to his shavetail son was: "Keep your bowels open and your mouth shut."

Good advice, if you can follow it without becoming a laxative addict! And that means if you can regulate your bowels mainly with what you eat instead of with medicines. Most medicines work by irritating your bowel so that the raw surfaces will weep and the extra moisture will wash bowel contents through. You feel almost as bad with laxative-disturbed digestion as you do with constipation. But natural food regulation ends all that. It gives you the benefits of an unclogged, almost gas-free system without the disadvantages of a drug-ravaged intestine.

If you have needed laxatives or enemas in the past, you'll probably have to start with a two or three week bowel-soothing program. During this phase, you can eat freely of meat, dairy products, eggs, and bread. Take two or more servings of fruit or juice each day, from the following list:

> lemon, orange, grapefruit (include one of these each day); bananas, pears, peaches, peeled apricots, baked apple, strawberries.

Also take at least two servings of bland vegetables every day, from this list:

> peas, string beans, carrots, beets, spinach, tomato or potato.

If you have headaches, indigestion, gas pains or more than a three day lag without a movement, take an enema consisting of one quart of warm water, one teaspoonful of table salt and two teaspoonfuls of baking soda for temporary relief. Detailed directions are given on pp. 130-132.

After your bowel has had a rest from harsh laxatives (or right at the start if you have never used them), add more moist-bulk producing fruits to your diet. The milder ones are:

> stewed prunes, cantaloupes, honey dew melon, raisins, currants, applesauce, plums, cherries and berries.

Somewhat more irritating fruits add effectiveness, but should be tried with caution since they cause some people extra gas pains and distress. Figs and dates are the main members of this group.

While you improve your intake of moist-bulk producing fruits and bland vegetables, you can also aid your bowel function by drinking plenty of non-alcoholic liquids—eight glasses or so a day—and taking mild daily exercise, such as a twenty minute evening stroll. In most cases, you will find these measures quite sufficient to keep your intestinal tract well toned up and open.

THIS CHAPTER'S TEN RULES FOR NATURAL FOOD INVIGORATION.

You can almost certainly win greater and longer-lasting vigor by choosing your meals and snacks according to these simple rules:

1. Depend on natural food, not pills or potions, for your vitamins, minerals and other bodily supplies.

2. Count food groups—meat, vegetables, fruit, dairy and grain—to fulfill all your needs instead of just your appetite for fuel.

3. Reach for a count of 4-5-5—four food groups in the morning, all five in the afternoon and evening—with sound mealtime choices.

4. Eat often for energy. Midmorning and midafternoon snacks measurably improve your power to get things done.

5. Choose snacks to fill your food group count as well as for quick energy alone. A completely filled 4-5-5 count works as a time-bomb tonic to make you feel better, stronger and more energetic inside a couple of weeks.

6. Eat more reserve-energy-supplying protein, in the form of lean meat if you can afford it, but also in the form of inexpensive egg, dairy and vegetable products.

7. Replace most stomach-slowing table spreads and shortening-rich piecrusts with protein-rich cottage cheese or meat and quick energy carbohydrates.

8. Dodge chemically treated fats (and cut down on solid

animal fats) for long-term tonic action. Mountains of research link these products with hardened arteries and accelerated decline into "old age."

9. Eat foods in a form you can readily chew, so that your body gets full advantage of them. Chew starches with special care instead of letting them slide down.

10. Regulate your bowels the natural way, with moist-bulk fruits, bland vegetables, fluids and exercise, instead of raking your intestine with harsh laxatives.

CHAPTER SEVEN

Liquid Refreshers and Natural Health Aids

An oriental myth tells how a holy man named Bodhidharma vowed to stay awake for nine whole years. After a valiant effort, he drifted off to slumber only three years later. To punish himself for his broken vow, he lived in the wilderness upon berries and leaves. In the process, he stumbled upon the means of brewing tea. With its aid, he made a second attempt and stayed awake for nine years after all.

When you need a lift, a refreshing cup of tea may make all the difference. Don't just say: "But I don't like tea." If the usual variety doesn't appeal to you, literally dozens of flavor combinations are available, ranging from light to dark and from fragrant to tart. Tea servings range from the Russian variety, so loaded with cloves, fruit juice and sugar that the underlying tea flavor is hardly distinguishable, to Chinese unseasoned pure. All varieties contain lift-giving caffeine and theophylline—the same ingredients sold in pill form as stay-awake stimulants. And all varieties are easy to prepare: if you have boiling water and something to drink from, you can have a cup of tea.

Of course, several other drinks give something of a lift. A cup of coffee contains more caffeine than the most widely sold nonprescription pep-up pill, and more than a cup of tea (which gets a little extra kick from its theophylline, however). Cola drinks have about half the stimulant content of coffee, besides quick-energy-fuel sugar. And cocoa contains a similar ingredient called theobromine, which usually perks you up without greatly affecting your later desire for sleep.

On the other hand, each of these agents does more harm than good in some people. Tea contains constipating tannins, which can knot up your bowels if you prove subject to their harmful

action. Coffee makes some people nervous and sometimes inter-
feres with sleep. As few as three or four cups of coffee each day
over a period of weeks occasionally causes indigestion, gas pains,
or constipation. Cocoa seldom causes complaints, but aggravates
any tendency toward overweight because of its high calorie
content. You have to choose the right stimulant drinks *for your
own system* and use them properly to perk up very often without
suffering harmful effects. Here's a helpful approach:

If you undergo sleeplessness, keyed-up feelings, indigestion, constipation or other complaints which might stem from
either tea or coffee, switch to cocoa, hot bouillon, or some other
caffeine-and tannin-free drink for three weeks. Complaints due
to your beverage habits will disappear. You can then resume tea
or coffee in small quantities. Gradually allow yourself more and
more until you find out how much you can take without immediate or long-term difficulties.

Rotate among several perk-up drinks instead of using
only one. You might take coffee in the morning, tea in the afternoon and cocoa in the evening, or take one of these beverages at
home while drinking a different one everywhere else. The harmful effects of one perk-up drink don't add up with those of another, so that you cut down the harmful action of each by
substituting a different one for part of your intake. Also, the
loss of effect which often follows continual use of one stimulant
does not cut down the action of its chemical cousins, and variety
helps to keep all of these agents working well for you.

Serve most of your perk-up drinks between meals, not
at table. You'll find that meals themselves give you a fresh head
of steam even if you keep stimulants to a minimum, while midmorning coffee and midafternoon tea give you a lift when you
need it. One cup of beverage helps round out the meal, but you'll
probably get more help without risking harmful effects by saving
seconds and thirds for a separate occasion.

If coffee and tea upset your digestion or your bowels and cocoa doesn't give you much kick (or pushes up your weight), try maté. Maté is a Paraguayan cousin to tea and coffee which is at least as stimulating without harmful effects on your digestion. You can obtain it in most good dietetic food shops, and brew it like tea. You'll acquire a taste for maté much more easily if you take tiny sips far back into your mouth, which puts its aromatic goodness near the palate and keeps its bitter after-taste away from the most sensitive portion of your tongue. Paraguayans sip it piping hot through tiny metal straws, but short plastic ones work equally well. Paper straws won't work, because the heat melts off their waterproofing wax.

Don't cancel out pep-up action with alcohol. Brandy and certain other alcoholic drinks make some people feel better after a tiring day by dulling their awareness of fatigue. However, alcohol slows body processes rather than stimulating them. Its action on fatigue is almost exactly the opposite of caffeine's, which speeds body processes and increases general awareness. The two approaches just don't work together, and you have to choose one or the other.*

Replace some perk-up drinks with drugless stimulators like bouillon, which we'll consider next.

DRUGLESS STIMULATING DRINKS

When a Minnesotan comes in after shoveling his walk, he expects to find a steaming hot beverage waiting for him. A luke-warm pot of coffee falls utterly flat—and for good reason. The caffeine or other druglike stimulant actually accomplishes only part of a hot drink's perk-up action, and mostly the long-delayed part at that. Caffeine or theophylline take half an hour or more to soak into your system. Whatever perk-up effect you enjoy

* This argument applies only to effect on fatigue. Alcohol and caffeine share mood-lifting effects, and do not particularly work against each other in building party spirit.

immediately after a hot drink stems from its temperature and consistency rather than from its stimulant content.

These non-drug effects probably accomplish more than the specific stimulants. One experiment proved that most people find lukewarm milk soothing and hot coffee stimulating, even when the caffeine has been removed from the coffee and added in double doses to the milk. Tasty steaming liquids like hot buttered rum and hot toddy have long been known as stimulants even though they contain alcohol, which has precisely the opposite drug-type action. Even hot water, perhaps with a little lemon juice, has long found favor as a perk-up remedy for victims of cold, influenza and post-virus fatigue.

Any steaming hot liquid can perk you up, whether or not it contains druglike stimulants. This approach proves especially apt in the evening, when coffee or tea often interfere with sleep. And the beverage need not be alcoholic—in fact, it usually proves more stimulating if it contains no spirits at all. You'll find all of the following varieties easy to fix, pleasant to take from either coffee cup or bowl, very tasty and refreshing:

Plain chicken or beef bouillon. Just boil water as if you were fixing tea, pour it over a bouillon cube in your usual cup, stir for a few moments and start to sip.

Seasoned broth. Boil beef or poultry for use in other dishes and save stock. Cool to allow ready removal of excess fat, and season with garlic salt, cracked pepper and thyme, or with your own favorite flavor aids. Store in refrigerator for use as above, or freeze in a refrigerator tray until hard, transfer the resulting cubes to an ordinary freezer box and thaw one portion at a time as needed.

Onion soup. Prepare from dried powder according to package directions, and sip steaming hot from a cup or bowl. Or prepare a simple variety by making beef bouillon as above and adding half a teaspoonful of onion salt plus a sprinkle of Parmesan cheese.

Next time you have guests in the evening, serve bouillon or broth instead of offering only coffee and tea. You'll be surprised at how many people prefer a product which can't possibly interfere with sleep or digestion, contains too few calories to threaten any waistline, and still gives a real lift along with its taste treat. And after you've served it a few times, you'll find it so refreshing and so little trouble to fix that you'll be fixing it for yourself several times a week. Or follow famous singer Leontyne Price's lead and carry a thermos with you almost everywhere you go.

DIGESTIVE TONICS

Next to general perk-ups, the most valuable use of natural health aids usually proves to be improvement in the workings of your digestive system. From the first stirring of appetite to the final disposal of wastes, every step of the digestive process can be improved by natural tonics. Without getting into the care of ailments or disorders,* let's see what drugless vegetable remedies can do:

Improved appetite. Strong and pleasantly sharp flavors stimulate your taste buds and increase the flow of gastric juice, improving both your appetite and your digestion. Many old-fashioned remedies, from chamomile tea to gentian root, use this principle to good effect, even though they have no drug-type action. Some of my most-plagued indigestion patients have obtained real relief from prescriptions mixed with cardamom compound and peppermint water, for instance, when pleasant-tasting compounds with the same "active" ingredients had failed utterly. A great many victims of run-down condition, people who can't get back on their feet after a virus infection, or otherwise healthy but "appetiteless" old folks find that bitters help them a great deal. Without some such simple aid, poor appetite leads to poor

* My book, *A Minnesota Doctor's Home Remedies for Common and Uncommon Ailments,* has separate chapters on indigestion. constipation, and rectal complaints.

eating, poor eating leads to continued weakness, and weakness leads to inactivity and still worse appetite.

Perhaps the easiest bitter to obtain these days is Angostura, which contains considerable gentian in a rather pleasantly-flavored base. Most supermarkets and almost all liquor stores handle Angostura, because many popular cocktails use this compound as an ingredient. Orange bitters, obtainable in the same places, also works effectively. A quarter to half a teaspoonful of either in half a glass of cool water often proves effective. Sip slowly fifteen or twenty minutes before a meal.

Strong unsweetened lemonade made turgid with grated lemon peel also may prove an effective appetite-improving bitter. You will find this more pleasant to take if thoroughly chilled. Half a glassful sipped slowly fifteen or twenty minutes before a meal usually spurs the appetite. Unfortunately, this mixture often proves too strong for people with a tendency toward acid indigestion or ulcer, and you should not use it if you have such inclinations.

Medicinal preparations which stimulate appetite without any risky drug-type action include cardamom compound and peppermint water. Although many drugstores do not carry these "old-fashioned" preparations in stock, they are relatively inexpensive even on special order. A teaspoonful of cardamom compound in half a glass of water, with or without ten drops of peppermint water, will often perk up your appetite before a meal.

Finally, sherry wine deserves mention. Three ounces of a dry, light sherry sipped slowly before mealtime definitely increase the flow of gastric juice and improve appetite. Unless you oppose the use of alcohol, you might find this a pleasant aid to appetite and digestion.

Digestion. Everybody likes to sit back and relax for a few minutes after a good meal. But if you sit back because you *have* to—because you feel dull and logy or uncomfortably full—then you ought to do something about it. A simple digestive tonic may help you to feel more sprightly and act more spry during the socially-crucial hour or so after meals, especially when the passing years have slowed the flow of your own digestive juices. Don't use digestive tonics for full-fledged indigestion, of course—they're meant to perk up body processes, not to combat ailments or disease. But use them promptly and as often as necessary for somewhat sluggish digestion.

Better digestion of starch often helps old people, people who cannot chew their food well because of poor teeth, and people whose mealtime hour is always rushed. Starch digestants convert hard-to-digest starch into quickly-absorbed, energy-boosting sugar-type compounds. This not only relieves after-meal gas and bloating due to poor starch digestion but also often improves your after-dinner energy and vigor.

 Among the natural food products, malt soup extract probably helps starch digestion most effectively. You can find this material in the infant food section of most drugstores. Two rounded teaspoonfuls sprinkled on breakfast cereal or suspended in water and sipped throughout lunch or supper works very well.

A medicinal tonic named Taka-Diastase also works effectively for many people. You can buy it without prescription in most drugstores. Try a teaspoonful in half a glass of water sipped before and during each meal, especially if bread, potatoes, noodles and other starchy foods sit like a lump of lead in your stomach after meals.

Sometimes starchy foods sit perfectly, but meats seem to digest quite sluggishly. If the problem hits mainly after fat-heavy fried foods or pork, biliousness or gall bladder trouble may be at fault —disorders calling for strong remedies rather than mild tonics. But protein-spurred digestive sluggishness sometimes yields to a simple switch to papaya juice as a beverage. The enzymes in papaya help to soften and digest meat particles—tenderize them right inside your stomach. You'll need to order papaya juice from a health food store rather than a grocery or drugstore and

sip it throughout the meal, but if slightly sluggish protein digestion has impaired your enjoyment of eggs and meat, you'll find
the effort quite worth while.

Bowel action. You can usually promote regularity without
bowel tonics. Drink plenty of fluids. Eat at each meal a moist-
bulk-holding fruit, like stewed prunes, cantaloupe, honeydew
melon, raisins, currants, applesauce, plums, cherries, berries,
apricots, pears and peaches. Choose bland vegetables like peas,
string beans, carrots, beets, spinach, tomato or potato, over cab-
bage and its heavy-fibered cousins. Take a twenty minute walk
each day to meet your need for activity.

If further help seems necessary, one natural tonic adds moist
bulk pleasantly and gently: psyllium seed, also known as plan-
tago. Suspend the seeds in orange or prune juice, or mix them
with a little hot water and spread the resulting gelatinous mass
on bread or other food. A tablespoonful of seeds once or twice
a day usually suffices, but larger amounts are harmless and smaller
quantities often do the trick. The seeds soak up 270 times their
own volume in water, making movements softer and easier to
pass. To provide this extra moisture, you must drink much more
water than when not using this tonic—at least three more glasses
a day.

Corn oil also acts as a mild bowel tonic. It works especially
well for slightly constipated children, who can usually get away
from need for harsh laxatives by taking a teaspoonful or less of
the oil each day. For this purpose, use the drugstore variety
instead of that sold in groceries for cooking purposes. Most
drugstores carry corn oil (U.S.P.) and can sell it to you without
a prescription.

THIS CHAPTER'S SUGGESTIONS FOR USING LIQUID REFRESHERS AND NATURAL HEALTH AIDS

Tea, coffee, cola and cocoa contain perk-up ingredients. You
can take full advantage of them without suffering harmful effects

by replacing agents which are doing you harm, varying your stimulant drinks, and using perk-up beverages during between-meals energy lag rather than at table. Some people find maté a good stimulant, especially if coffee and tea upset digestion. In any case, don't supplement perk-up beverages with alcoholic ones—the two work at cross-purposes in this respect. If you need further pick-me-ups beyond your personal coffee-tea-and-cola limit, try either cocoa or steaming hot clear soup—bouillon, seasoned broth or onion soup—for a real and completely harmless lift.

When some people want a tonic, they really need perk-up mainly for appetite, digestion or bowel action. If appetite needs a boost, try bitters, lemonade with grated peel, cardamom, or sherry. For better starch digestion, malt soup extract or Taka-Diastase often help. Moisture-bulk-providing diet, psyllium seed and corn oil aid bowel action without the harshness of full-fledged constipation remedies.

CHAPTER EIGHT

Internal Cleansing
for Attractiveness,
Comfort, and Health

In my Johns Hopkins days, the fresh-scrubbed steps of Baltimore's row houses always impressed me. Even in the slums—most since replaced by neat apartments—filth might lie in piles within the hallways, but the front steps gleamed.

You might think such step-scrubbing vain or foolish, but it represents a basic human trait. All of us tend to combat difficulties which *show,* and try to ignore less outwardly-noticeable problems. We wash our faces several times a day while letting unwholesome, discomfort-breeding crusts pile up inside our noses. We polish our front teeth carefully while food particles between our grinders promote bad breath and tooth decay. We scrub relatively harmless grime off our hands while suffering in silence through the miseries of a waste-clogged rectum or irritated female organs. Such preoccupation with externals is human nature, but it's still worth combatting. A few minutes a week devoted to internal cleanliness can make you feel tremendously more comfortable and refreshed. From top to bottom, here's how to keep your body's crypts and crevices comfortably clean.

NOSE

A plug or crust inside your nose can cause considerable misery. It blocks off breathing, irritates your nose lining, and pulls uncomfortably on imbedded hairs. You almost can't help picking at it, often causing a sore nose, nosebleeds or other damage. Moreover, the very presence of the crust shows that your body's barrier against cold germs and other infections has been impaired.

118

You'll feel much more comfortable and often prevent colds and other miseries by keeping your nasal passages clear.

Humidification. Inside your nose, tiny sweeper cells move a thin blanket of sticky mucus back into your throat at a slow but steady rate. If you can keep the mucus and its underlying sweeper cells from drying out, this mechanism will take care of almost anything that lodges or forms inside your nose, including plugs and crusts formed from the mucus itself. Any particle which lodges in this mucous blanket moves back and is swallowed inside six minutes.

In warm, moist weather, the inside of your nose keeps itself spanking clean, because its mucous blanket never dries out. But air holds less moisture as it grows cooler—about half as much for each five degree temperature drop. When you heat air in the wintertime without adding moisture to it, dryness soon congeals bits of your mucous blanket into crusts and halts sweeper cell action.

You can keep your body's own cleansing method working by adding moisture to any heated air you breathe. Unfortunately, it takes a lot of moisture—literally gallons each day for an average Northern U.S.A. house. But your nose will benefit from whatever steps you can take. You'll find several suggestions in Chapter Ten (pp. 158-161).

Anointment. If you can't keep your house humid enough to prevent dryness and crusting, or if you spend a lot of time in a dry-air heated office or shop, nasal anointment proves a great comfort. A small dab of lanolin or unmedicated petroleum jelly every day keeps your nose's sweeper cells hard at work. You can buy either of these materials at any drugstore without prescription. Place a dab the size of a matchhead on the tip of your finger or on a Q-tip and deposit it on the wall between your nostrils about half an inch inside your nose. The sweeper cells will spread it as body warmth makes the glob melt. **Children**

under twelve and victims of bulbar polio or other diseases affecting the swallowing mechanism should not use this method, since immature or damaged swallowing muscles occasionally allow even thick ointments to trickle down into the lungs.

Snuffling, sprays and irrigations. When material accumulates anywhere in your nose—crusts near the nostrils, thick mucus which narrows the breathing passage, or globs of drainage continually tickling your throat—you may need to take stronger action to clear your nasal passages. However, the action you take should never cause further damage. You should avoid nose-blowing, for instance. It drives germs from the nasal passages up into the sinuses and ears, causing many miseries and illnesses. Best stick to techniques which work without interfering in any way with your nose's normal self-cleansing mechanisms or with its soundness and health, like snuffling, bland sprays and irrigation.

Perhaps the simplest way to clear your nasal passage without blowing or picking is by snuffling. Cup your hand slightly to make a hollow in its palm. Fill this hollow with lukewarm tap water. Sniff the water up into your nose, then let any surplus run back into your washbasin. If one side of your nose is much more clogged than the other, you may need to plug the more open one by pressing on the side of your nose with your finger or thumb before you can draw water up into the clogged nostril. If the sniffed-up water stings or burns, your town's tap water probably has a lot of chlorine in it. You can eliminate the problem by letting your snuffling water stand overnight in an open vessel so that the chlorine evaporates.

You may need a more lasting "moisturizer" than ordinary tap water if your problem includes thick drainage down the back of your throat. Most such post-nasal drip and tickle actually does not result from real disease. Irritation from smoking, from dry air or from dust simply makes the mucous glands work hard and fast, while excess dryness thickens the material into sticky globs. These cling in the back of your throat while you swallow again and again. A little extra moisture thins the mucus so that it passes on down into the stomach at the first swallow, which turns "post-nasal drip" into perfectly normal irritant-disposal. You can make a fine moisturizing spray right in your own home by using this recipe:

> 1 tablespoonful of glycerin (available at your drugstore without prescription)
> 1½ tablespoonfuls rubbing alcohol
> 1 teaspoonful table salt
> 1 pint water

Let the water stand in an open vessel overnight if it has a chlorine odor. Mix the ingredients and store in a corked or capped bottle.

You can spray the inside of your nose several times a day with this solution as necessary, using a plastic atomizer which you can get from your drugstore for half a dollar or less. You'll find that one or two squirts soften crusts and thin mucus so that the sweeper cells can clear out your nose in a hurry, and leave a thin protective coat that lasts for hours.

If moisturizing spray fails to keep your nose clear (which happens mainly during the thick-mucus phase of a cold or a sinus attack) irrigation usually proves the best way to clear your nasal passages. A fountain syringe, available in most homes for giving enemas, works very well. Use a clean or freshly boiled outlet tube, and attach the glass portion of an eyedropper to its end for a tip. Clamp off the outlet tube or bend it double and pinch it off. Dissolve two level teaspoonfuls of table salt in a quart of lukewarm water in the bag. Hang the bag so that the water level is 12 to 18 inches above the level of your nose, and lean over a washbasin or sink. Point the glass tip straight in, not up toward your forehead, and insert it half an inch or so into your nostril.

Hold your finger against the side of the nose to seal the nostril against the sides of the glass tip. Hold your breath and allow the solution to flow into your nose. It will flow back out through the other nostril without running down your throat. Cut off the stream before you need to take a breath, open your mouth and satisfy your need for air. Hold your breath and repeat the irrigation. When the solution is about half gone, switch the tip into your other nostril and reverse the direction of irrigation. Continue until the solution is gone or the nose entirely clear.

EARS

Your ears normally form quite a bit of wax which coats the inside of the ear canal. Any dirt, insect life or other material which gets into your ears sticks in this coating. When you chew your food, motion of the jaw milks the wax and trapped soilage out of your ear canal. Like your nose's mucous blanket, though, ear wax sometimes dries out and accumulates. Dry wax causes considerable discomfort, itching, impaired hearing, and upset stomach (because the same nerves supply both parts of the ear canal and the digestive organs).

You can avoid all these problems by keeping your ear wax from drying out or by removing accumulations when they occur. Unless you must keep fluids out of your ears because of a perforated eardrum or constantly draining ear, these procedures are completely safe.

Ear anointment. Ear wax is chemically a heavy oil, and softens up when mixed with lighter cousins. Sweet oil has been used as a wax-softener for centuries, and works effectively (if rather slowly). Warm the oil in a teaspoon by applying the flame of a match underneath. Test on your earlobe before putting into the ear, to avoid burns.

Modern oil-and-water ointments work faster than plain oil, since the oil they contain is supplemented in its action by the chemicals which keep the oil and water from separating. Hydrophilic ointment (U.S.P.) or a preparation of boric acid in a cream base (such as Borament) works quite well. Either can be obtained in any drugstore without prescription. Apply a small amount in the ear canal while lying on the opposite side, and remain in that position for several minutes until the material warms to your skin and spreads.

Dishwashing detergent. Only a small amount of soap or detergent can get at a lump of wax inside the ear canal. Soap solutions have never proved strong enough to either dissolve a lump of wax or cause any admixture of wax-softening water. However, liquid dishwashing detergents frequently allow water to soak into the wax plug. Three or four drops of detergent to a teaspoonful of warm water allowed to soak in for five minutes or more at least three times a day usually makes dry wax work out of the ear inside three days.

Special wax-softening detergents. Several wax-softening agents such as Cerumenex are available in your drugstore. A few people react badly to these agents and get skin eruption from them, so they should be used only if other methods fail.

Ear irrigation. Even when dishwashing or special detergents fail to work alone, they usually soften wax enough that it washes free quite easily. Use water which is as hot as is comfortable, testing it on the lobe of the ear and in gradually increasing little squirts. Use a one-ounce all-rubber ear syringe from your drugstore. Pull the ear backward and slightly downward to straighten out its canal, and squirt gently toward the upper part of the canal's back wall. The tip should never be inserted far enough to block off free flow of water from the canal, which allows dangerous pressure to build up. If the wax has not come loose after using a pint or so of water or if discomfort in the ear, dizziness, or nausea occur, best enlist a doctor's aid. Never try to scrape the wax out—the eardrum is paper-thin and very easily damaged by hairpins or similar objects.

THE MOUTH

You can frequently sweeten your breath and make yourself feel fresher by mouth cleansing. Before you start, though, check yourself for these non-mouth sources of bad breath, most of which call for special remedies:

Foul-smelling sinus discharge, for which nose irrigations give temporary relief and a physician's care often proves worthwhile. Sinus headaches point toward this source.

Smoldering infection of the lungs or bronchial tubes, which you should strongly suspect if a phlegm-producing cough accompanies foul breath.

Protein digestion which forms malodorous breathed-out wastes. This disorder causes no other complaints or difficulties and has no serious effects on health, but is very hard to combat. The breath smells like rotting flesh even when there is no sinus drainage and the mouth is clean and healthy. A sharp change in diet often helps, whether proteins, fats or carbohydrates are increased. To increase proteins, take cottage cheese, eggs, fish and meat in large quantities at each meal. To increase fats, take two tablespoonfuls of cooking oil before each meal. To increase carbohydrates, take two slices of bread with each meal. Each program deserves a two-week trial before settling on the one that works best. Take care to keep a well-rounded diet, and to adjust your food intake to keep from trading bad breath for a weight problem.

Gum brushing. When bad breath actually starts in the mouth, decaying food particles between the teeth or infection of the gums and tooth sockets is usually at fault, and better tooth and gum care often gives permanent relief. For odor-free breath and a trouble-free mouth, concentrate on brushing your *gums* rather than your teeth. Gum-brushing prevents or cures many infections in tooth-supporting structures and sockets. These conditions otherwise cause more misery and lost teeth, as well as more mouth odor, than all other dental disorders put together. Since you can't brush your gums without getting food particles out of the crevices near the base of the teeth, gum-brushing also prevents cavities much more effectively than ordinary toothbrushing.

You need a small-headed toothbrush to get at your gums properly. Two rows of bristles work best, cut to form a level surface without tufts or arching. Stannous fluoride-containing toothpaste might help if you have much trouble with cavities, but almost any dentifrice works well in combatting bad breath and supporting-structure disease. You can fight breath odor by brushing at any time of day, but after-meals timing adds to cavity-fighting action.

Gum-brushing tries to milk pus and infection out of the tooth sockets. Each stroke therefore starts near the base of the gum and swipes toward the tooth's biting edge. A rolling action with the wrist and fingers usually does the job most easily. Pressure should be firm but not harsh. Brush the gums inside as well as outside of the teeth. Ten strokes in each area gives ideal massage, and usually cleans out any food particles caught between the teeth at the same time. If your gums get sore after brushing, the problem is usually that you brush downward along the tooth so that the brush picks up the gum fold at the rim of the tooth socket. Lifting the brush entirely free of contact on each return stroke so that all rubbing is toward the tooth crown usually allows prompt healing.

Breath sweeteners. For temporary relief while trying other measures or as a last resort when nothing else works, you might try Alkaline Aromatic Solution N.F., obtainable from any drugstore without a prescription. Thin it with an equal volume of warm water and use as a mouthwash. Tincture of Myrrh N.F. also works fairly well and is more concentrated, so that you can carry a small bottle in your pocket or purse for use at work or during social engagements. Ten drops in half a glassful of water makes an effective odor-dispelling mouthwash. A teaspoonful of baking soda, ¼ cup of peppermint water and half a glassful of tapwater makes a good mouthwash, too.

Sucking lifesavers or mints several times a day sometimes gives relief by letting sugar-digesting bacteria overgrow the protein-digesting ones which cause most odor. However, this program increases cavity formation, and is unwise for people who need frequent fillings. Sucking cloves or odor-killing lozenges may help temporarily.

THE FEMALE ORGANS

A great many women need an occasional douche to avoid body odor, especially a week or so after menstruation (when the glands at the mouth of the uterus form extra mucus through which sperm can swim with ease). Daily douching removes juices whose strong acids normally act as germ-destroyers, and may make you slightly more subject to minor infection at the mouth of the womb. Somewhat less frequent douching does no harm, though, especially if you use solutions which match the normal vaginal juices in acid content. Moreover, you need only an occasional douche to keep you clean and odor-free if you use ideal technique.

Equipment. A fountain syringe (gravity-fed bag type) works much better than a bulb syringe (squeeze type). Use the largest comfortable tip to avoid any risk of threading your douche instrument into the mouth of the womb by mistake. Ladies without sexual experience must often use a rather small tip, and should therefore insert it three inches or less to avoid the womb's opening.

Solutions: For ordinary cleanliness, one tablespoonful of white vinegar to a quart of lukewarm water works well. Another satisfactory mixture contains ten drops of lactic acid (U.S.P., available in any drugstore) to a quart of lukewarm water. Most commercial douche powders are expensive, hard to mix, and have no advantage over plain vinegar.

Preparation: Mix the solution in your syringe bag, and suspend so that the water level will be about three feet above the tip when you are lying in the bathtub.

Lubrication: Use a little K-Y Jelly, glycerine or Crisco to make insertion of the tip entirely comfortable.

Insertion: The adult-sized tip is usually blunt-ended with several openings along its sides. It should be inserted until all openings lie within the vagina. A virgin can often insert a douche tip more comfortably if she lies down with back, hips and knees almost on a level and introduces the douche tip along the front surface of the vagina.

Controlling flow: Let the solution begin to flow. Using the sides of both index fingers, press the folds at either side of the vagina together so that they seal off the opening and allow the water pressure inside to expand the vagina. This process opens up all the folds and creases in which secretions otherwise stagnate. When the vagina feels somewhat tense, release the fluid in a gush and allow solution to flow freely for a few seconds. Stop up the opening again and allow the solution to expand your vagina again. Continue until solution is exhausted.

Cleansing and protection to heal minor irritations. Mild itching or discomfort at the female opening usually comes from minor irritation. You can eliminate some common causes of difficulty, like inadequate drying after urination and soil-conveying forward-wiping after bowel movements. Careful drying of all folds with soft facial tissue and dusting with baby powder or cornstarch helps urine-scalding. Cleansing after movements with only one front-to-back motion for each fold of toilet paper also prevents problems. If these measures do not suffice, or if slight leakage of urine when you laugh or cough seems a factor, Diaprene ointment (from the baby counter of your drugstore) may help.

If ordinary cleansing fails, try Burows' Solution, which you can also buy without prescription. Mix three ounces to a quart of lukewarm water for a soothing, healing douche. If irritation lies close enough to the surface to allow application of cotton pledgets or soft cloths wet with the medication, two ounces of Burows' Solution to one pint of water works well. Many women also get relief from Tucks, which are small medicated pads meant to be tucked between folds at the female outlet and available without prescription at any drugstore.

Frequent irritation, irritation accompanied by watery discharge or bleeding, irritation which gets worse after each menstrual period or irritation severe enough to cause any swelling deserve a doctor's care.

Douches to encourage pregnancy. Even in couples with a normal capacity to reproduce, the sperm cell operates under a severe handicap. To start a pregnancy, it must find its way through body tubes and passages whose length is tremendous in proportion to the sperm cell's size. The odds against the sperm cell multiply if it must swim part of the way through strong acids. Women who want to become pregnant may find their chances improved by acid-neutralizing douches.

Acid-neutralizing douches help mainly during the "fertile period"—the two or three days on either side of the fourteenth day after the start of menstruation. Take them inside half an hour before intercourse if possible—certainly inside an hour. Three tablespoonfuls of baking soda in two quarts of lukewarm water work very well. Two tablespoonfuls of baking soda and one tablespoonful of table salt in two quarts of water is also satisfactory.

Do not use acid-containing douche powders or solutions while trying to conceive. While such materials are not sufficiently hampering to be worth-while aids in preventing pregnancy, they may possibly tip the balance in borderline situations.

Douches in conjunction with birth control. Since directions for using various birth control preparations often mention douching after intercourse, many people think that prompt douching prevents pregnancy. This is totally false. Many sperm find their way almost immediately into the mouth of the uterus, beyond which douches cannot reach.

Most birth control methods work best when chemicals remain at full strength and devices remain undisturbed for several hours. The directions "douche after four to six hours" might better read "*Don't* douche for at least four hours, then douche if necessary for the sake of cleanliness and comfort." An ordinary vinegar or lactic acid douche works perfectly well.

Relaxing tub-douche before marital relations. Women sometimes find sexual relations difficult due to nervous tension or the physical effects of a recent, rough encounter. A tub-douche combination often relaxes and soothes them sufficiently to make satisfactory relations possible.

Tie a long string to the douche bag and loop it over the shower-curtain rod so that the bag can easily be filled without leaving the tub. Take a leisurely hot soak in water at about 94-98 degrees (measured with a candy thermometer). After you feel thoroughly relaxed, fill the douche bag with hot water at about 112-118 degrees. Insert the tip under the water and douche, using the usual technique. Adjust the water temperature to the hottest level you find comfortable. Do not douche at this temperature unless sitting in at least four inches of water. The vagina will stand considerably warmer water than the surrounding skin, and run-off may cause burns unless cooler water quenches it.

Alum douches. Especially after childbirth has stretched their tissues, some women find their husband-pleasing ability somewhat improved by alum douches. One teaspoonful of alum to two quarts of lukewarm water makes a suitable solution. Aluminum acetate, available at any drugstore without prescription, has a similar action in the same strength solution.

Douches after relations. Douches after satisfactory sexual intercourse give little benefit unless necessary for cleansing. If failure to reach a satisfactory climax leaves discomfort and congestion, a douche with one teaspoonful of alum or aluminum acetate solution to two quarts of cool water (about 75 degrees) often gives relief.

BOWEL

Here in Minnesota, spring lasts from when the trees leaf out until you start to perspire. It's one of our most beautiful seasons, but it sometimes lasts only fifteen minutes. So we don't have a lot of time for spring tonics, and try to keep fairly well cleaned out all year long. Nature's main bowel aids—fruit with each meal, plenty of water to drink, and daily exercise—usually do the trick. If these measures fail, a properly-given enema gives prompt, thorough and entirely comfortable relief.

If enemas have seemed unpleasant to you in the past, you've probably followed one or more outmoded technique or idea. You don't have to "hold back until the urge builds up." That just makes you endure extra discomfort. You don't need bowel-irritating material like soapsuds or turpentine, which lead to griping pains and cramps. You don't even need to run in the solution rapidly to stretch the bowel wall. Just follow these directions:

> Choose the smallest enema tip, or use a soft rubber catheter in place of the enema tip if the area has proved overly sensitive. Keep your leftover slivers of soap soaking in a little water and use this soap jell as a lubricant. Its action just inside the rectum stirs an active urge toward bowel movement without the griping you get from a full soapsuds enema. Mix four teaspoonfuls of baking soda and two teaspoonfuls of table salt with two quarts of warm water in the enema bag, keeping the outlet tube firmly pinched off or clamped. Hold the tip above the water level in the bag and release the outlet tube. Lower

the tip slowly so that the solution runs out into the tube and pushes out all air. Clamp or pinch off the tube.

Suspend the enema bag so that its water level will be about eighteen inches above the tip's outlet. If possible, attach it by running a long string across the top of a smooth shower-curtain rod or similar hanger which will act like a pulley and allow you to raise or lower the bag without getting up. Lie on your left side with your right knee resting opposite your hip and your left leg as straight as is comfortable. Reach across your body with your left hand and lift the right buttock out of the way. Insert the enema tip or catheter with your right hand. Do not insert any farther than necessary to keep it in place— extra tubing only coils around in the rectum and does not make the enema any higher.

Raise or lower the enema bag so that the solution runs in slowly and does not create any sensation of pressure or discomfort. If cramping or uncomfortable fullness develops, stop the flow by bending the enema tube over on itself or clamping it, and take two or three deep breaths. You may also need to massage the left lower abdomen with the flat of your hand—not with your fingertips, which may cause bruising when you knead the deeper tissues. Most such discomfort comes from spasm in the bowel wall: if you have difficulty of this sort, use spasm-soothing hot water rather than warm water for future enemas. About 110 degrees (measured with a candy thermometer) is safe and effective.

Whenever you feel that you have had enough, cut off the flow of solution. You probably will not need the entire two quarts—most people get good results with two or three pints. Remove the enema tip and expel the material as soon as the impulse hits: there is no need to hold back until the urge builds up. The soap jell used for lubricant washes out promptly during passage, so that later griping or irritation seldom troubles you with this technique. If such aftereffects should occur, however, you can soothe them quickly by slowly injecting into the rectum one ounce of Amphogel liquid (an antacid stomach-soother available anywhere without prescription), using an infant syringe or all-rubber ear syringe. Restrain any urge to pass this material if possible, and after a minute or two you will feel entirely comfortable.

THIS CHAPTER'S ADVICE ON CLEANSING
BODY CRYPTS AND CAVITIES

You feel much more comfortable and refreshed when your body's crypts and cavities are clean.

Your *nose* has its own cleansing system, with a mucous blanket to snare dirt and sweeper cells to move it back where you can swallow it. Humidification keeps this natural cleansing system working. Anointment with petroleum jelly or lanolin also helps. Snuffling, moisturizing spray and irrigations help you to clear out clogged passages or persistent "tickle" without harmful blowing, picking or throat-clearing.

Your *ears* normally form soft dirt-catching wax which chewing motions milk out continually. When the wax dries into chunks, you can soften it with sweet oil, hydrophilic ointment or Borament. Dishwashing or special detergents also help. Properly softened wax usually works its way out of the ears without further action, but an extra-hard plug sometimes must be washed out.

A clean *mouth* contributes to sweet breath and a fresh feeling. Check yourself for common outside-the-mouth sources of bad breath before resorting to mouthwash. Brush your gums instead of your teeth, and use breathsweeteners if necessary.

The *female organs* often require occasional douches to keep clean and odor-free, although daily douching is unnecessary and unwise. Irritation frequently disappears with improved cleanliness, Burow's Solution douches or compresses. Acid-neutralizing douches may encourage pregnancy, but no safe form of douche will prevent conception. Relaxing tub-douches sometimes aid in preparation for marital relations. Alum or aluminum acetate douches may aid husband-pleasing potential. Cool alum douches often relieve congestion after an unsatisfying episode.

Properly given enemas clean out your *bowel* as comfortably and conveniently as any laxative, with a great deal less constipation-aggravating action. Follow the detailed directions given here for entirely comfortable relief of temporary irregularity.

CHAPTER NINE

Extra Vigor and
Energy Through
Bone-Balance

Campers in the Minnesota woods use about twelve guy ropes when they pitch a center-pole tent. I wonder how many ropes they would need if each center pole were cut into 29 blocks of wood, each balanced precariously on its neighbor beneath, and how long it would take to put up such a tent. It wouldn't be very efficient, would it? Yet that's exactly how your skeleton works. Taking each bone or rigidly-connected group of bones as a unit, your leg, spine and skull have 29 freely movable pieces. To make matters worse, your bones aren't normally arranged in a straight stack. They arch forward in your low back, backward across the chest, and forward again in the neck.

Dozens of muscles work constantly at guying up this floppy, crooked stack of freely-movable bones. Better bone-balance can almost certainly save you lots of energy, helping you to get through the day with greater strength and vigor.

SELF-TRAINING

Unlike most tonics and refreshers, which benefit you only for a few minutes, hours or days, a single concentrated effort to improve your poise and balance may benefit you for the rest of your life. Once new patterns of body balance become firmly fixed, you can forget about them. You won't fall back into less efficient ways.

Bones stacked straight up on one another take less effort to support than bones stacked at angles. Your self-training program concentrates on decreasing the curves and tilts of the spinal column, particularly in the low back and neck. Although these curves are often perfectly normal, your body still operates more efficiently if you can flatten them somewhat. Two simple exercises help:

1. Walk away from a wall. The child's name of this exercise, "paper doll," gives a graphic picture of it. You try to plaster yourself against a wall like a sheet of paper, then walk away without changing the alignment of your spine. The details:

> Stand with toes pointing straight ahead, feet about four inches apart, and heels about four inches from an unbroken, flat-surfaced wall or closed slab door. Lean back against the wall or door and plaster the palms of your hands against it about six inches away from your hips.
>
> Try to bring the hollow of your back as close as possible to the wall. Roll your hips under and tighten them in a kind of burlesque bump. If properly done, this motion should make the buttock muscles hard and firm while leaving the upper part of the body in unchanged relationship to the wall. Pull your stomach up and in. Lift up your chest (not your shoulders) toward the ceiling. Try to perform these motions without tightening the muscles of the upper abdomen: the lift should come from the chest muscles and the muscles below the umbilicus. If you find this difficult, take several deep breaths while relaxing the upper abdomen to restore free movement.
>
> Next, flatten your upper arms and shoulders back against the wall. In trying to do this, you will draw your shoulderblades nearer to your spine and flatten the curve of your upper back. Try to get the "feel" of this position, which you should maintain when you walk away from the wall even though your arms and shoulders then relax.
>
> Next, force the back part of the crown of your head up toward the ceiling. This motion should straighten the curve at the back of your neck and draw your chin in toward your voicebox. It balances your skull's weight on the top of your nearly-straight spine.
>
> Now rock forward away from the wall without altering the position of your hips, back or neck. Walk with your toes still pointed straight ahead. Let your arms fall with-

out allowing your shoulderblades to wing out. Keep the back of your head always pushing up toward the ceiling.

Repeat the whole procedure every time you catch yourself slumping back into a curved-spine posture. For the first week or so, this might mean a few moments backed against a wall each and every time you stand on your feet, or at least eight or ten times a day. Two or three reminder exercises a day might suffice for the next two or three weeks, after which the new patterns will be so thoroughly entrenched that you will continue them without any deliberate effort.

2. Sit flatfooted and tall. You probably spend almost as much time sitting as standing, which makes the way you balance your body on a chair important to your energy. Moreover, a slumped sitting posture can hamper circulation to and from important organs. For instance, one group of women whose work involves constant sitting lost more than twelve days a year from menstrual cramps. Posture chairs and a set of sit-straight exercises cut their time loss to three days each year, showing that three-fourths of their previous suffering stemmed from posture-caused congestion in the female organs.

You can reach the ideal sitting position by using a wall to align your spinal column, then sitting down without changing your back's position. Go through this procedure a few times until you get the feel of bone-balanced sitting. From then on, you can simply run through five self-commands whenever you feel that your body balance has sagged away from the ideal:

Feet flat on the floor.

Stomach pulled up and in, but with upper portion fairly lax.

Chest (but not shoulders) lifted.

Shoulderblades drawn somewhat toward spine.

Back of head's crown pushed up toward the ceiling.

Like ideal standing habits, better sitting becomes automatic after a few weeks of frequent self-reminders. You'll enjoy its benefits of extra vigor and improved health for many years. Why not make a brief but concentrated self-training effort, starting today?

Straightening sidewise tilts. Nobody's two sides match each other exactly. Slight assymmetry does no real harm, unless it throws your body out of balance. Even then, your body automatically adjusts: but its adjustments throw an extra burden on certain joints and muscles, cause pressure on certain blood vessels and nerves, and make you less efficient and less comfortable. A few moments spent checking for sidewise slants, and an hour or two devoted to their correction if present, may save you a great deal of energy, prevent almost daily nagging backaches, and considerably improve your appearance from this moment forth.

Mirror tests. You can easily test yourself for sidewise tilts with a mirror hung on wall or door, a carpenter's level (if you have one handy) and an eyebrow pencil, lipstick or piece of soap. Undress, stand in front of the mirror, and notice about where the reflection of your hip bones falls. Using the carpenter's level if available, draw a straight line across the mirror at this point. Stand barefooted with your thumbtips resting on corresponding parts of your two hipbones. Relatively lean people have no difficulty locating the bony prominence at the upper end of the thigh bone. Plumper ones can use the two "front corners" of the bony brim which separates the flank area from the hip. Move toward the mirror or away from it until the reflection of your thumb-marked hip areas falls exactly across the line you previously drew on the mirror. You will be able to tell at a glance if one hip lies higher than the other. Follow the same procedure with somewhat higher-placed lines to determine whether your shoulders and your eyes are level.

Leg length equalization. If your hips tilt, the reason is almost always that one leg (usually the left) is shorter than the other. Stand with a deck of playing cards under the shorter leg's heel and check hip levels once more. Add or take away cards until you find the exact thickness which makes your hips level. Usually you will feel considerable relief of strain on the back muscles and ligaments when your hips are level and your spine straighter. Measure the thickness required, and have your shoemaker add corresponding extra height to your heel. The leather wedge he adds should taper slightly toward its front so that the front of the heel doesn't jut down too far. An ordinary heel wedge (which costs about one dollar) is not too noticeable with corrections under one inch, which covers almost all tilts except those due to old fractures or paralysis. Inside-the-shoe devices will correct much greater differences in leg length without noticeable assymmetry, but these are expensive enough to make doctor-checked measurements worthwhile.

Chest stretching. If hips are level but shoulders aren't, try stretching the short side of your chest. Sit sidewise on a straight chair with the low shoulder away from the chair back. Choose a chair whose back ends approximately opposite your nipples. If the chair back is too high, sit on telephone books or cushions to bring your body into the proper relationship. Stretch the arm from the shorter shoulder up over your head and touch its fingers to the opposite ear. Arch your body sidewise across the chair back, pushing the raised elbow over your head and toward the ceiling. You will feel the chair back pressing against one side of your body and the ribs stretching apart on the other. Continue the stretch for five seconds, then relax. Repeat five times at a session, about three times a day.

Eye leveling. If your eyes are slightly off level, leave the line drawn on your mirror. Each time you look in the mirror, stretch the back of your head toward the ceiling and set your eyes at the proper levels. Hold this position until it becomes a habit.

EQUIPMENT FOR BETTER BONE-BALANCE

An expert can balance his body weight on a rope or wire as easily as on the floor. But he has to concentrate on it continuously. In the same way, you can keep your bones balanced upon one another in perfect effort-saving array while perched on high heels or seated on a lounging chair. But more suitable equipment makes the job much easier and more automatic.

Shoes. Like the leaning tower of Pisa, fatigue-causing faults in body balance often come from a poor foundation. Men and women alike frequently gain new energy by supporting their feet in a poise-improving position. Miseries previously blamed on everything from neuralgia and arthritis to old age and overwork may also clear up with shoe-improved bone balance: slight shifts in foot position often change bony relationships to relieve pressure on ligaments, nerves and joints all the way up to the skull's attachment.

Sideward roll, not heel elevation, makes the biggest difference to bone balance. Men's "sensible-heeled" shoes fail to give the needed support almost as often as women's high-heeled ones. If your feet roll inward, your thigh must turn inward too, to save your knee ligaments from intensive strain. Try these motions yourself: Sit with both feet flat on the floor. Without moving the knee and thigh or lifting either the ball of the foot or the heel, raise the little-toe side of one foot off the floor. Keep the foot in this position and try to straighten out the knee. If you can do it at all, which most people can't, you'll feel considerable ligament strain. Next, put both feet on the floor and raise the little-toe side of each. Keep your feet in this position and stand up. You can do it, but only by rolling your thighs inward so that your kneecaps point more or less toward each other. This throws a strain on your hips which you can only relieve by rolling your pelvis backward, making your buttocks and abdomen protrude unattractively and your low back turn into a sagging, muscle-supported curve instead of an energy-saving column.

A pair of foot-supporting or foot-tipping shoes can prevent or reverse all these shifts: At the very least, they will help you maintain bone balance which is already good. If weak arches, swaybacked stance, neuralgic pains, low back discomfort or round upper back have troubled you, foot-tipping shoes may make you look and feel years younger.

A shoe which provides a new foundation for your body's stack of bones must hold your heel and arch firmly. Such a shoe often rebalances your weight without further modification. If wedges or other devices are needed, snug foot-supporting shoes keep the feet from turning back to the old position inside the tipped shoes. Either way, you need shoes with certain structural features, fitted precisely to your feet.

> *Selecting shoes.* Check two points regarding shoe structure:
>
> 1. The firm heel-gripping cup built into the shoe should be too stiff to dent readily with your thumb, and should extend forward at least to the mid-arch.
>
> 2. The narrow part of the shoe sole underneath your arch should be reinforced with a stiff steel shank. Test for rigidity by placing the shoe on a level surface and pressing down firmly on the inside of the sole just in front of the heel. If the back end of the heel lifts up, the sole is too flexible.

A number of companies make suitable shoes for foot-tipping modification, both in "practical" and stylish fashions. Among them are:

> Men: Florsheim (custom long-counter* models only), I. Sabel, Thompson, Smith Syncroflex, Wright Arch Preserver (long counter models only).

---

* Shoe manufacturers use the term "counter" to signify the shoe's heel-gripping cup.

Women: Miller Foot Defender, I. Sabel, Selby, Matrix, Drew.

Children: I. Sabel, Child Life, Pied Piper.

Heel height. Men do not need to worry about heel height or style, since fashion matches practicality. Most women need one pair of high heels for dress-up occasions. However, low or medium heels give much better stability and support. You will probably find that the hip-slimming, back-straightening, chest-lifting action of properly fitted foot-tipping shoes does more for your appearance than slightly higher heels. If wedges or other foot-tipping devices are necessary, low or medium heels almost always give enough benefit to both appearance and vigor to make them worth while.

Checking fit. When you find a store which carries suitable shoes, you need to be sure of getting a proper fit. Don't depend entirely on the shoe salesman. Check every pair of shoes point by point before you buy.

First, check *arch length.* The ball of your foot should fall exactly opposite the sharp inward curve at the front of the shoe's arch. Toe-room makes very little difference to shoe support (although it affects comfort, corn formation and so on). Only arch length, which determines whether the front of the shoe shank spreads your weight to the front part of the foot bones, really makes a difference. Ignore the ends of your toes as long as they feel comfortable, and check the ball of your foot to determine proper length.

Second, check *front foot width* across the bases of your toes. Stand with your weight on one foot. If the shoe top either pinches your foot or bulges out beyond the margin of the sole, the shoe is too narrow. If the leather buckles easily when you try to pinch up slack from side to side, the shoe is too wide.

Third, check *heel width.* Raise up on your toes and let your weight back down on your heels several times. If your heel moves inside the shoe, its back segment is too wide.

If your feet differ somewhat in size (which is true of many perfectly normal individuals), fit the larger. If you cannot find shoes which fit your entire foot, fit the arch length and front-foot width correctly and have your shoemaker put in a set of molded heel counter inserts or tighten the heel.

Wedges? When you get your pair of foot-supporting shoes home, make one further test. Tie a paperclip to the end of a piece of thread. While standing comfortably on both feet, hold the thread against the center of one kneecap, letting the paper-clip dangle so that it barely touches the top of your shoe. Repeat on the other side. If this test shows that the line of gravity falls slightly toward the outer margin of each foot, you do not require any special wedges or devices to improve bone balance (although if you are bowlegged, wedges which raise the outer portion of your heel may decrease joint strain on your knees). If the paper-clips touch toward the inner margin of your foot, wedges or other foot-tipping devices will prove of considerable help not only to foot comfort but to body mechanics. Slight inward shift of the weight-bearing point—to the center of your foot's side-to-side dimension or perhaps ¼ inch beyond—calls for ¼ inch wedges to raise the inner margin of your heel, which any shoemaker can fit at quite modest cost. Marked inward shift—more than ¼ inch inward from the foot's center—calls for half-inch heel wedges, which in turn throw so much strain on the shoe's shank that a plastic arch support or heel-to-arch-front reinforcement is neces-sary. You will usually need to visit an orthopedic appliance dealer, brace shop, or orthopedic shoe specialist to get this type of equipment. With extreme weight-bearing shift, especially if accompanied by flat feet, painful feet or knock knees, special shoes made to an orthopedist's specifications may be necessary —an expensive proposition, but one which often gives relief from fatigue, spinal curvature, backache and a dozen other problems you would not suspect of stemming from your feet.

Picking-up-the-carpet walk. When foot-tipping shoes prove helpful to bone-balance, most people find that even a few steps taken in the old, tipped-out position may interfere with the benefits. Men and women who have felt "old before their time" from aches and pains, numbness or neuritis brought on by pressure of displaced bone and overly-tense muscles may lose all the advantage of wearing special shoes simply by walking to the bathroom and back in their bare feet or in soft slippers every morning. For such people, a simple exercise helps a lot: simply roll your feet inward as if trying to imitate a bow-legged cowboy, curl your toes as if trying to grasp the carpet pile with them, and walk on the outer borders of your feet. If you get in the habit of doing this whenever you stand up without your foot-tipping shoes on, you will enjoy much greater benefits.

Which shoes when? My wife keeps a small plastic bag in her capacious purse. When we go downtown together, she usually wears low or medium heels and carries her fancy pumps in the "satchel." If she decides to try on dress clothes or go to a restaurant for lunch, thirty seconds in the powder room puts her in high fashion. The rest of the time, she enjoys the extra comfort and staying-power of sound, foot-supporting brogues.

Whether you go so far as to carry extra shoes with you or not, a pair of comfortable foot-supporting shoes at home and at the office can probably help you to establish and maintain proper bone-balancing poise. It only takes a moment to change your shoes. Instead of slipping them off, switching to slippers, or wearing old shoes which give you no support, why not switch to foot-supporting low or moderate heeled shoes? You'll look better, feel better and stay vigorously energetic longer at virtually no cost in money, time or effort.

Rugs and pads. The first time I visited a General Mills

industrial plant. I was somewhat surprised to find each worker's station equipped with a smooth-surfaced, yielding pad.

"All the comforts of home," I remarked to the superintendent who was showing me around.

"Right," he replied with a grin. "Anything for the worker. As long as it pays off in production increase."

He went on to explain that men who worked on a yielding surface not only felt less footweary by the end of the day, but also accomplished more.

"They finish the day strong," he said. Which is exactly what you want to do, too—finish the day with energy left over to keep on doing the things you *want* as well as the things you *must*. A cushioning rug or floor mat in areas where you often stand can help a lot.

Chairs. Twenty-six of your twenty-nine bone segments still remain precariously balanced on one another when you sit down. A well-chosen chair gives a sound foundation for a proper sitting pose, which saves you a great deal of energy. Check for these qualities:

1. Seat height. When you sit with both feet flat on the floor, your thighs should rest comfortably along the chair seat without undue pressure at its edge. You can adjust for a too-low seat with a cushion or foam-rubber or tufted pad. If you sometimes wear high heels and sometimes wear low ones, try to fit seat height to the low heels and keep an inch-and-a-half to two-inch cushion handy for use with high ones. A chair with too high a seat can sometimes be salvaged by using a small, thick throw rug underneath your feet with its edge in front of the chair's legs.

2. A molded or contoured seat. If your chair is going to steady you in bone-balancing posture, you have to sit on the same spot every day. A chair with contours into which you settle your weight-supporting parts fulfills that need. The contours needn't be fancy: a wooden-seated kitchen chair often has exactly the amount of hollowing required. Simply avoid flat-surfaced or non-contoured chair seats, or fit a contoured seat pad over them.

3. Back support. If you have a true posture chair, you can adjust the back so that it presses firmly against your ribs just beneath the lower margins of your shoulderblades when sitting straight. Otherwise, make a special pad to get similar support from an ordinary straight-backed chair.

> Buy a piece of denim, canvas, or other sturdy cloth eight inches wider than your chair's back and twice its length. Hem both sides to make a pillowcase-like cover for the chair's back. Put the cover inside out onto the chair's back, sit upright in the chair, and mark the level at which the lower margin of your shoulderblades strikes. Cut a foam rubber pad 2 inches thick, six inches from top to bottom, and slightly narrower than the chair's back. Cut another piece of cloth large enough to bridge this pad. Sew this piece of cloth to the inside of the chairback cover just below the shoulderblade-margin marks. Place the rubber pad just below this seam. Draw the cloth down over it and sew to the chairback cover in such a way that the rubber pad remains firmly in place. Turn the chairback cover right side out and slip in place over the chair's back with the pad toward the seat. Sit in the chair to test pad placement: if properly made, the cover should hold the rubber pad against the back of your chest just beneath your shoulderblades. Attach cloth tapes to the sides and bottom of the chairback cover as necessary to hold it snugly in place.

Stools. For up-and-down jobs, whether in the kitchen or in the workshop, a high stool saves your energy. A normal-height chair wastes more work by making you lift your body weight whenever you get up than it saves by aiding bone balance. When you'll be sitting most of the time, a stool slightly lower than your hip-level with a foot rest or rail works best. For continual up-

and-down tasks, choose a stool which matches your hip level so closely that you can slide on and off with no effort at all.

By actual measurement, you can save about one-third of the effort you would otherwise spend in a machine shop or on ironing and meal preparation with a proper-height stool. Wouldn't you enjoy having that much extra energy left over after your chores are finished?

Hammocks. When you rest on a hammock, you do more than re-invigorate a weary stack of bones by temporarily unstacking them. You stretch tight muscles to reverse the swayback curve. A pillow or two under your knees increases the effect, and a small pillow or rolled towel under your neck (not under the back of your head) may increase your comfort.

If you want to use a hammock in your office or shop, you can probably attach one end to the inside of a closet with extralong rope. For use, swing out into the room with the extra rope length transversing the closet. For storage, detach the far end, roll back into the closet and slide onto an empty shelf. A sturdy spring clip on the hammock's room-end rigging and a fixed (but possibly hidden) hook lets you set up or collapse the unit in a few moments.

You can get similar action from a very firm bed or couch by lying on your back with two pillows under each leg. Arrange the pillows so that your lower legs are parallel with the floor and your knees are slightly bent. In this position, the bed presses up on your hips and shoulders while the weight of your trunk presses your low back toward the ground. A soft mattress impairs this action by coming up to meet your trunk. Extra-firm bedding—either an orthopedic mattress or an ordinary cotton one with a piece of plywood underneath—increases the effect.

A few minutes' hammock- or bed-borne break helps a lot, especially if low back curvature causes you to tire out or develop backaches every afternoon. Some workmen eat lunch in a hammock, some housewives hang one near the telephone. One way or another, you can almost certainly arrange a refreshing back-muscle-stretching flop several times a day if you find that it adds substantially to your vigor and comfort.

EXERCISES

Simple self-training, aided by proper equipment for standing, sitting and lying comfortably sometimes fails to improve bone-balance and poise. Then weak muscles in some areas or overly tight ones in others usually prove at fault.

Your abdominal muscles have a great deal to do with bone balance in your low back. Although these muscles seem like only thin sheets by comparison with the heavy back muscles, they use the entire rib cage and the entire pelvis as wrenchlike levers to increase their effectiveness. If your abdominal muscles are somewhat weak and your back muscles overtight, you cannot straighten an extra spinal curvature by simple self-commands. You must strengthen the abdominals and stretch the back muscles before self-training has any chance of success. Such a program takes extra effort, but it also brings extra rewards. Correcting a considerable bone imbalance yields more extra energy and comfort at the end of each day than correcting a mild one. Not to mention improved appearance: corrective exercises for substantial curvatures usually make your body look much more lithe and attractive, improve the fit of your clothing, and aid your poise.

Straightening the low back. Decreasing curvature in your low back can make you look less hippy, nip in protruding buttocks and flatten your abdomen. It also gives the rest of your spine a level foundation upon which to stand, squares off round shoulders and corrects hollow chest. You save a tremendous amount of energy by straighter carriage, too, since low-back curvature forces your trunk muscles to support much of the upper body's weight. Especially if you can't straighten your spine sufficiently to plaster its whole length against a wall when doing the "walk away from a wall" procedure (p. 137), a few simple exercises often make you look and feel 100 per cent better.

Curl-up back stretch. Lie on your back with hips and knees flexed, grasping both legs just below the knees with your hands. Pull your knees up under your chin as far as possible. Hold for five seconds. Relax to first position for three to five seconds. Repeat ten times.

Head lift. Lie on your back with feet separated and drawn up close to your buttocks, knees together. Simultaneously raise your head and flatten your low back against the floor. Hold for six seconds, breathing normally to be sure that upper abdomen remains relaxed. Return to first position for several seconds and repeat five times.

Elbow twisting. Start from same position, but with fingers laced behind your neck and elbows thrown well back. Raise your head, flatten your low back, and turn your head and arms to one side. Keep the elbows thrown well back. Return to center and turn toward the other side. Return to center, let your head drop back and relax to starting position. Repeat five times.

Buddha sitting. Sit on the floor with the soles of your two feet flat against each other. If your proportions permit, clasp both hands around your joined insteps: otherwise grasp both legs or ankles as far down as you can comfortably reach. Simultaneously press both knees down toward the floor and draw your shoulders down and back (so that the shoulderblades pull in toward the spine). Hold this position of tension for five seconds, then relax for a few seconds. Repeat five times.

Squaring up the back and shoulders. If you have a round back, drooping shoulders or a hollow chest, there's a very good chance that corrective exercises can make you look better and feel more youthful. Many of the aches and pains, numbness and minor discomfort which people blame on "old age creeping up" actually stem from sagging muscles and bones which press against nerves or blood vessels. Corrective exercises often end all that.

Of course, nobody wants to put effort into stretching exercises if they aren't going to do any good. You should always straighten any excessive hollow in your low back before starting on the upper areas, or work on both at once. A hollow low back forces you to bend your upper spine forward to keep your balance, and keeps corrective exercises for round back from doing any good. If you have a barrel chest from long-smoldering lung or bronchial troubles such as asthma or chronic bronchitis, exercises will never square up your back. A spine frozen with arthritis or extreme old age will not yield to home correctives. The type of hollow chest in which the breastbone seems caved in beneath the level of adjoining ribs stems from faulty bone structure rather than from posture, and will not yield to exercises. Round back from bone-weakening diseases like tuberculosis or from severe injury cannot usually be altered. In most other situations, stretching and exercise have enough chance of success to be well worth a trial.

Ground-hugging. Lie down with a rubber kneeling pad or foam rubber cushion under the rounded area of your back. Bend your knees to a comfortable position, resting both feet flat on the floor. Flatten your low back and neck as close as possible to the floor. Fold your hands together behind your neck, press your elbows to the floor, and take a deep breath. Let the breath out and relax both your back and your arms. Repeat five times. Now flatten your low back and stretch both arms overhead, trying to touch your fingers to the floor as far away from your scalp as possible. Bring your hands down to your sides and relax. Repeat five times.

Buddha sitting. This exercise, described on p. 150 for use in excess low back curvature, also helps rounded upper back. It is especially apt when both conditions afflict you.

Stall bar stretch. If you have access to a YMCA or other gymnasium, you'll probably find it equipped with stall bars—smooth wood rails hung across an otherwise unbroken wall at six to eight inch intervals. Stand on tiptoes with your back toward the stall bars. Reach the highest one possible and lift yourself up until part of the weight is off of your feet, then bend your knees to increase the pull. Be sure to *lift* rather than just bend your knees and hang limp. The shoulderblade muscles must be tense while you are hanging to give any benefit.

If you do not have access to stall bars, you can rig up a one-man equivalent sufficient for this particular exercise in your garage, attic or basement. A few lengths of two-inch dowel or lead pipe nailed across the space between adjoining studs will do the trick. Be sure one piece falls at a level where you can just reach it by standing on tiptoes, and that other pieces fall every six to eight inches in the area where your head, chest and hips strike. Or simply put a crosspiece every eight inches from floor to ceiling, especially if several members of the family might use the apparatus.

CHAPTER NINE'S BONE-BALANCING TECHNIQUES

Keeping your floppy, crooked stack of freely-movable bones erect costs you a lot of energy. You'll add substantially to the strength and vigor available for other things if you improve bone-balance.

A few weeks of *self-training* often give lifelong benefits in increased energy and bodily comfort. Learn bone-balance by walking away from a wall. Keep yourself flatfooted and erect when seated. Use mirror tests for sidewise tilt, and correct it with heel wedges, rib stretching or eyeleveling exercises.

Special items of *equipment and furniture* often improve energy-saving bone balance. Foot-supporting or foot-tipping shoes give a sound foundation for ideal carriage. Long counters, rigid shanks, and low or moderate heels improve support. Check shoe fit with regard to arch length, front width and heel width. If the paperclip-dangling test shows poor weight distribution, have your shoes (or at least the ones you wear for on-your-feet-occasions) fitted with foot-tipping devices. A cushioning floor pad or rug conserves energy, too. Posture chairs or home-padded equivalents can save you considerable effort. A high stool for up-and-down jobs conserves energy. Hammocks actually help to stretch tight, curvature-increasing back muscles, as well as to provide rest. A firm bed with special pillow arrangement can do the same.

If all else fails, you can often achieve energy-saving, contour-improving ideal bone balance through *exercises*. Straighten excess curvature in the low back with the curl-up back stretch, the head lift, the elbow twist, or with Buddha sitting. Square up round upper back and shoulders with ground-hugging, Buddha sitting, and hanging from stall bars.

CHAPTER TEN

Breathe in Refreshment

Turn a city couple loose near a North woods lake, and you'll soon see certain changes in them. New energy, new appetite, new contentment with each other and with the world. Wonderful effects of exercise, beautiful surroundings—and pine-scented outdoor air.

What air does. Everybody knows that you need good elimination to feel your best. Yet people who would never think of letting wastes accumulate in their intestinal tracts neglect their most important form of minute-by-minute elimination— disposal of noxious wastes in the breath. The Black Hole of Calcutta and several other disasters have proved that rebreathed air can prove downright deadly, even if enough oxygen is provided. Even in ordinary situations, repeatedly rebreathing the same air can lead to lassitude, headache, muddle-headedness, and many more serious effects. Certainly you can't feel your best unless a constant flow of air carries away breathed-out wastes.

Air also affects your response to coldness and to warmth. A few simple steps help you to winter well—to stay healthy, feel comfortable, and remain efficient at work and play. Spring fever and summer lethargy both respond to air-involving tonic and refresher techniques.

The air around you provides oxygen, of course. Ordinarily you can forget all about that function, though. You can't exhaust the oxygen in indoor air as fast as air exchange through chinks and openings replenishes it. You don't need to make any deliberate efforts to supply fresh oxygen in your home or office.

156

AIR IN COLD WEATHER

A Minnesotan quickly learns some tricks for keeping warm, both outdoors and in. He likes to brag about his heartiness and warm-bloodedness, so he doesn't think of his cold-weather habits as survival skills. But scientific studies have shown that anyone, even a far-North Eskimo, freezes from about the same exposure. Minnesotans can keep warm in a blizzard and enjoy a hearthside evening without feeling a draught because of what they *do,* not what they *are.* Anybody can achieve the same results by following their patterns of winter living.

Keeping warm outdoors. Minnesota warmth-assuring stunts depend on three scientific facts: Here they are, with the simple techniques you can use to apply them:

1. Heat rises. A snugly buttoned coat collar with a soft scarf to seal any leaks saves a tremendous amount of body heat, which otherwise pours out of your coat's neckhole like smoke from a chimney.

2. You lose a lot of heat through your lungs. Every breath of air which you draw into your lungs enters cold and leaves warm. Heat lost in this way has more to do with body cooling than that which works its way past warm clothing, especially if active exercise makes you breathe heavily. Old-timers fight this loss in extra-cold weather by arranging a scarf into a breathing tunnel in front of their faces, so that the breathed-out air helps to warm and moisturize the breathed-in.

3. Cooling of blood on its way to hands and feet has a lot to do with their coldness. Mittens and overshoes help a lot, but long underwear or extra sweaters often accomplish even more.

Summer breezes versus winter draughts. When you measure air movement indoors, you find that many draughts which cause real discomfort move slower than the mildest summer zephyr detectable by your skin. Even at exactly the same temperature, the same speed of air movement can feel like a caressing breeze or a gooseflesh-raising blast. Yet outdoor air has no special ingredient, and indoor air no marked deficiency. The difference comes down to one crucial quality: moisture content or humidity.

So-called "gooseflesh" results from the tiny muscles in the skin which pull the hairs upright. Exactly the same action which protected our monkey ancestors against loss of heat and moisture by pulling their fur erect still follows exposure to either cold or dryness. It causes equal discomfort no matter which condition brings it on.

Moisturizing home air. The teakettle boiling merrily on the back of a Minnesota cookstove serves more purposes than one. It's ready for instant hospitality, with the drip coffee maker standing by. And it also moves a steady flow of moisture into the air. When folks warm up in a Minnesota kitchen, they really *feel* warm. Literally gallons of water boil away into the air each day in an old-fashioned kitchen, helping to keep our hearty housewives healthy.

Not that lots of our farms aren't modernized. And homes, too. If they're *completely* modern, they even include humidifying systems to boil away gallons of water again and make the heated air more comfortable and healthful. Every Minnesotan knows that extra air moisture definitely lowers sensitivity to draughts and keeps you feeling better through the winter months, besides helping to ward off colds, nose troubles and sore throats. The same facts apply in milder climates, although perhaps to a less obvious degree.

Push down that thermostat! A great many people who complain of draughts suffer from *too much* air-drying heat instead of *too little* warming action. Warm air can hold more vaporized moisture than cold. Whenever you heat air an extra five degrees, you double its capacity for moisture. If you have added no new moisture, the same amount of wetness is spread twice as thin, and the air has twice as much drying action. A ten degree rise means fourfold increase in dryness. A fifteen degree rise multiplies drying power by eight. Unless you add moisture as you heat, indoor air thus becomes progressively drier as you push the thermostat up. I've seen many people, especially in the over-sixty age group, who "just can't get warm—get goose-flesh even when it's over eighty in the house," yet feel perfectly comfortable in moister air at seventy degrees. Often no extra moisture is required—just *decreasing* the temperature so that the moisture already present can do some good.

Humidifiers. You can spend a lot of money on humidifiers, but often the money is well spent. If you stay comfortable with the thermostat at seventy instead of heating the whole house to eighty all winter, your lower heating bills—and possibly lower doctor bills from decreased colds—will pay for a humidifier quite soon.

Whole-house humidifiers work by letting water evaporate in the warm air that emerges from your furnace. A unit which scatters the water into tiny droplets (which have vast surface in proportion to their weight) or drips it along easily-replaced filters usually works best.

Room or space humidifiers usually vaporize water in a sort of boiler and either blow it into the air or feed it through a tube in which it has a chance to cool. Since they heat the water by electricity, they usually cost more to operate than furnace-type humidifiers. However, they work well enough to let you humidify a room, apartment, or office in an unhumidified building.

Homemade air moisteners. Any arrangement that puts warm water where air circulates will increase humidity. If you have more time than money, you can provide these essentials at nominal cost. A homemade unit lacks the automatic water-feed and other features of expensive systems, and thus requires frequent refilling. But this involves no more work than watering your house plants, and quickly becomes an almost automatic part of household routine.

In houses with hot air heat, water pans just inside the registers work rather well. Rapid movement of still-warm air makes for lively evaporation, while the pans can be refilled more easily than units in the furnace cowl and no great harm is done if one overflows.

For vents which enter the room horizontally, remove the grill and measure the nearest level surface on which a pan can be placed. Any flat-bottomed low-sided pan will do—photographic darkroom trays, which come in a wide variety of sizes, work very well. A piece of plastic or rubber tubing taped into place with one end in the tray and the other protruding through the grill makes filling quite easy. Firmly attach the end of the tubing which sticks into the pan with its end about ¾ inch from the top so that you can use it as a fullness indicator as well as a supply tube. When filling the pan with the grill in place, pinch off the tube *while it is still full of water.* Lower the free end below pan level and release. If the water level in the pan is above the tube's inner opening, water will siphon back through the free end and you will know that the pan is full. If no water siphons back, pour a bit more through, then repeat the test.

If your registers come up through the floor, you can usually hang the water pan six inches or so under the grill, using ordinary baling wire. A funnel with a tube that fits between the grill fins (which may have to be bent slightly for the purpose) makes refilling easy.

Radiant heat offers less opportunity for easy humidification. Flat pans on steam or hot water radiators can take the edge off of dryness. A small electric fan greatly increases such a pan's efficiency if set to blow constantly across the water surface. Measures to spread moisture from clothesdrying and other water-vaporizing jobs through the house also help. Our Scandinavians put their lack of undue modesty to work by taking their hot baths and showers with the bathroom door open, for instance.

Bedtime ventilation. Probably the issue of whether the bedroom windows should be up or down has broken up few marriages, but it has put a great many under strain. Actually, fresh air has no real advantage over indoor air in an ordinarily spacious room, except for two qualities: it is cooler, and it causes air motion. With the windows closed, the room takes an hour or so to cool off after you turn down the heat. Meanwhile, the furnace stops working, and air circulation from your furnace fan or from the rising of radiator-heated air promptly stops. So the air hangs stifling still around you while you try to get to sleep, and you toss and turn instead of dropping off promptly.

Actually, you can usually solve the problem of bedroom stuffiness without the heat wastage of an open window. If you have forced air heat, you can probably turn on your furnace fan with the manual control intended for summer ventilation and let it run continuously. You can run an electric bedroom fan at low, quiet speed, either all night or at the bedtime hour with an automatic appliance timer. Another sound approach is to undress, then open the windows wide and close the bedroom door while performing your toilet. In five or ten minutes, the room will cool thoroughly. Close the window and open the door as you go to bed. The air movement from air warming near the walls and radiators will last long enough for you to get to sleep without any risk of chilling later in the night.

Clothing and cold walls. Although warm or cold air plays some part, the rate at which your body loses heat depends also on the warmth or coldness of surrounding walls and objects. This problem shows full-force in an unfinished basement, where cold walls and floors can make you feel quite cool even when the air is comfortably warm*. The overheated and therefore overdry air with which you then surround yourself makes you unhealthy. If you spend any appreciable time in a basement or other cold-walled space, you can improve both your comfort and your health by taking these steps:

If at all possible, keep heat from moving to the cold walls from your body with a wool rug, blankets hung along the walls and similar measures. One of my patients who suffered frequent colds, chilblains and gooseflesh blamed most of her trouble on the hours she spent in her basement doing laundry and ironing. An old set of drapes hung along the walls and an ancient wool rug in her ironing area helped a lot, even though the air temperature remained unchanged.

Dress to suit heat loss, not indoor temperature. On cold days, heat loss to cold walls and through windows may make you need an extra sweater or a set of long underwear to stay comfortable even if the room temperature is in the seventies.

When the walls and floors are so cold that you cannot stay comfortable even in heavy clothing without raising the temperature above 72, make a special effort to moisturize the overheated air. Better to make the walls sweat than to suffer the skin discomfort, nasal crusts, nosebleeds and extra colds or sore throats which dry air will impose.

COMES THE SPRING

If you put a smoldering cigarette or piece of string near a cold window in a heated room, you will find considerable air movement. Even if the window fits tightly, nearby air becomes colder, which makes it become more compact and heavy. This air sinks

---

* "Dank" or "damp" spaces have long been known to be unhealthy. Moisture on the walls causes no problem of itself, though: it merely shows that the walls are cold enough to cause condensation, and therefore cold enough to cause the chain of events here described.

toward the floor near cold spots, and pushes air upward in other parts of the room. Hot air rising from radiators and registers has a similar action in reverse.

Air moves constantly in a heated room on a cold day, but natural air currents almost disappear when the temperature difference between outdoor and indoor air lessens. Until the weather becomes warm enough to make you open the windows, air hangs almost motionless. **This stagnant-air interval coincides almost exactly with the time when most people feel logy, dull and listless from "spring fever."** Although lack of exercise in winter and other elements may have some bearing, sluggish air movement seems at least partially at fault. And an open window or a small electric fan often proves just the spring tonic you need to put you back on your feet—one of the cheapest and most pleasant invigorators you've ever tried.

AIR IN WARM WEATHER

When summer zephyrs blow, air serves new purposes in maintaining your vigor and comfort. Air can *cool your quarters* to reduce the actual warmth around you, and air can *cool your body* by evaporating sweat.

Night air as a coolant. You can knock six to ten degrees off the daytime temperature of any well-insulated building by proper use of night air's cooling action. Thoroughly airing the room at night leaves the walls and contents cool, as well as the air. If you close off the room, several hours pass before the temperature warms up to the outdoor level.

An attic fan aids this process by drawing cool night air through the building in vast quantities. An exhaust fan or large window fan also works well, especially in a building vacant at night (so that the noise and air blasts make no difference). Turn on your attic, exhaust or window fan at dusk, and open windows which will make the air pass through the entire space you want cooled.

With an attic fan, windows in all parts of the building can be opened. With an exhaust or window fan, nearby windows should be tightly closed, room doors left ajar and windows at the opposite end or corner of the building open wide. If you haven't any large fan, simply open all the windows and depend on natural air exchange. In any case, the windows should be shut as soon as possible in the morning. Draw the blinds (which should be quite opaque or backed with aluminum foil) to keep out solar heat, and use small room fans to keep air circulating. An indoor-outdoor thermometer also helps: as soon as enough solar heat penetrates to make the indoor temperature match the outdoor one—usually in late afternoon—you can open the windows and use your attic or window fan again.

Getting air to your skin. You can enjoy some of the effects which make lakeside breeze-bather feel soothed and invigorated even in a sweltering room or office. This sensation comes from *all-over ventilation*—gentle air movement caressing your whole body. You can't completely match it indoors or in clothing, but you can come reasonably close.

Compared with the usual table-top position, an electric fan placed on the floor gives more cooling and better air circulation. Tilting the fan upward allows it to blow cooler air up from near floor level. In most rooms, you can work out an arrangement which bounces the air off a wall to soften and broaden its stream into a gentle, all-over breeze. By unscrewing the oscillator so that the fan blows constantly in one direction, you can usually keep it working full force for your cooling and comfort. You'll also avoid the nasal congestion and sneezing which quite a few people get in response to the alternating air blasts and stuffiness of an ordinary fan-ventilated room.

In warm weather, air movement should reach every part of your body if possible. The switch from a clinging rubber pad to bare wood or plastic may help. Ventilation-aiding straw chair pads give further aid. Layers of clothing not in contact with your skin should be porous enough to permit air to flow through them readily. Layers of clothing in contact with the skin need not be porous if they are moisture-absorbent—cotton knit underwear and shirting actually act like wicks, spreading each drop of perspiration over a vast length of air-exposed thread and increasing its body-cooling evaporation.

BREATHED-IN REFRESHERS

Napoleon Bonaparte almost conquered Europe partly because he could work twenty hours a day. To fend off fatigue, he kept a small bottle with him at all times, but his bottle contained Eau de Cologne instead of the traditional brandy. Napoleon took *sniffs* instead of *snorts,* and found them most refreshing.

Eau de Cologne has no druglike action. However, scents link themselves quite readily with certain moods, actions and occasions, as every woman acknowledges in her use of perfume. Why not link a scent which you find agreeable with moments of relaxation? Dampen a handkerchief with a few drops of Eau de Cologne, shaving lotion, or other agreeable scent. Wave it gently beneath your nose while you follow one of the relaxation routines described on pages 80-86. After a few occasions, you'll find the scent thoroughly linked with relaxation in your mind. The odor itself will soothe your tensions, help you loosen up, and bring faster and more complete refreshment. Perhaps a similar effect explains why pine odor, which most Minnesotans associate with leisure-time activities, perks up our workers. Researchers have found this effect very real and measurable—both in increased output, decreased mistakes and improved satisfaction with their work.

Air fresheners. A breath of odorless air refreshes you more than a breath of stale or unpleasant-scented air. Air fresheners neutralize bad odors and give the air a mild, refreshing tang. While many people use these products to rid bathroom of odor, few think about air-freshening in a stale-smelling kitchen, office or shop where it could do tremendous good.

Air ions. Preliminary studies show that electrically charged particles present in the air affect your mood and efficiency. Positively charged particles make you feel logy and depressed, negatively charged ones brighten your mood and heighten your energy. Methods of changing air ionization seem somewhat impractical at present, and further research on their effects seems necessary, but you might watch for further developments.

THE GIST OF CHAPTER TEN

Besides providing oxygen, air helps your body rid itself of wastes and regulate its temperature. You'll feel better and stay healthier if you help it to perform those functions effectively.

In wintertime, outer clothing that fits snug around the neck, tunnel breathing, and long underwear help to conserve warmth. Indoors, you'll find that sensitivity to draughts comes from lack of moisture in the air, not from lack of heat. Lowering the thermostat sometimes helps, humidification with store-bought or homemade equipment always does. Need for fresh air at bedtime often comes from lack of air movement during the house-cooling phase, and may yield to a fan as well as to an open window. When cold walls or windows lead to heat loss, you need heavier clothing instead of overheated air.

To some extent, "spring fever" comes from lack of air movement. An opened window or small electric fan often helps.

Come summertime, you can use air to cool your quarters or to evaporate body-cooling sweat. An attic fan, window fan or exhaust fan helps you to use night air for cooling, although natural ventilation also works fairly well. A floor-placed, non-oscillating electric fan with its air stream bounced off a wall best mimics cooling breezes. Straw seat-mats and loose or wick-like clothing help evaporate the sweat.

In any season, you can gain energy and vigor through certain breathed-in refreshers. Eau de Cologne or air refresheners deserve your thought. Air ions offer interesting possibilities.

CHAPTER ELEVEN

Eye Easers for
Brain Vigor

A man with an outdoor job almost never suffers from brainweariness. Not that he doesn't use his brains: outdoor work can keep you thinking all the time. But he never reaches the state of muddleheadedness, tension and fatigue which afflicts many desk workers. He never suffers the plague-at-the-end-of-the-day which fills the city bars at quitting time, not with convivial celebrants but with quick shot-guzzlers seeking an alcoholic quietude to carry them through the homeward ride. He never finds his hours of freedom and family life plagued by the constant irritability of so-called brain fatigue, turning what should be pleasant hours into a constant struggle for self-control.

Our Minnesota tourist bureaus boost the virtues of the great outdoors as antidotes to this sort of thing. But outdoor air and scenery actually have very little to do with it. Most "brainweariness" really consists to a considerable degree of "eyeweariness"—the result of both deliberate and unconscious straining for clear vision. Eyeweariness comes partly from work your eye actually does in adjusting to brightness or dimness and to near vision or far. But most eyeweariness is caused by tension in your eye's musculature when such adjustments are impossible—when you must look at both bright and dim objects at the same time, or try to see clearly both near and far. You can do all the eye work you want without fatigue, if you eliminate the tension of eye confusion. Simple eye easers require little or no effort, but with their aid you can banish tired eyes, eyestrain complaints, and dullness, irritability or fatigue from close eye work, paperwork or reading.

170

LIGHT VERSUS CONTRAST

A dozen times or more while you were growing up, your parents probably told you, "Turn on the lights before you ruin your eyes."

Now modern science has found that often as not the right command would be: "Turn *off* the lights before you ruin your eyes. Or at least make the lighting softer to relieve your eyes of strain!"

Unless the whole room is moderately bright, extra light on your book or newspaper only increases the contrast between it and other areas within your range of vision. *Contrast* rather than *dimness* causes most eyestrain and fatigue.

Subject lighting. Your eyes work better for close work and reading fine print in rather bright light *if the background is almost as bright*. However, extra light does not make it easier for you to see objects for which the light is already adequate. Brightness equivalent to that from a bare 100 watt bulb at three to four feet lets you read ordinary print with minimal strain. Even for very close work, extra-fine print and reading scrawled handwriting the bulb at two feet gives sufficient brightness. Brighter light makes reading no easier. In fact, it usually does more harm than good by creating unavoidable glare and excessive contrast with dark furniture, floors or corners.

Scattered and bounced light. Direct light from a single source makes harsh shadows, which add to eye-fatiguing contrast.

You can test your reading area right now for too-direct light. Spread your hand six inches in front of this page. Are your finger and palm shadows black or light gray? If they are black, every shadow in your range of vision confuses your eye's regulating system by signalling for darkness-vision settings. That's why a properly scattered and bounced light lets you keep on reading or working for extra hours without becoming "brain-weary," and usually proves very helpful to desk workers, executives, students or pleasure-readers, and anyone who does close eyework.

Sources of softened light. If you need new lamps or fixtures, your lighting problem can be easily solved. Large translucent lampshades make for diffuse lighting. Indirect fixtures or opal bowls bounce light from small sources off vast stretches of ceiling or wall. If you want help with selecting suitable lamps, write to your state society for the prevention of blindness (in your state capitol) or call the home service department of your local electric company for pamphlets and other materials. For very fine work, bluish light works best, but for ordinary reading and handiwork the color makes no difference.

Unfortunately, most people can't afford to revamp their whole house or office lighting system. Unless you're due for such purchases, anyway, you may find these methods more practical:

Foil caps or backward-shining bulbs. If you want more diffuse lighting, you usually need bigger lightbulbs to make up for the light lost and spread around the room instead of concentrated on your reading. Larger lightbulbs demand an arrangement which shields your eyes from direct rays, scattering or bouncing them off of a substantial area. Foil-capped or backward-shining bulbs often prove the perfect answer, making the *reflector* rather than the *bulb* the room's light source.

I used to work in an unfinished basement. Indirect lighting simply wouldn't work because of the dusty, nonreflective floor joists that made up the ceiling. But a large saucerlike reflector cost me only a few cents from the mail order house. A lightbulb with a silvered front end that threw all its light backward against the reflector let me triple the light available without excess glare.

A lamp with an opal bowl intended to bounce part of the light off of the ceiling and let the rest through as a soft glow can be made to direct more of its light downward by fitting it with a bulb with a silvered end. This is especially desirable when the ceiling and walls are too dark or far-distant to reflect indirect light.

If you want to use up large but unsilvered lightbulbs which you already own, or if you need bulbs silvered on the side, foil caps may be the answer. Ordinary aluminum foil molds to a lightbulb to form an efficient backward-bouncing light reflector. Be careful not to get it too close to the socket, and secure it in place with dabs of nonflammable cement.

Fluorescent lamps give fairly diffuse bright light which often works out well in lighting desks and work tables. A mixture of fluorescent and ordinary light is probably better than straight fluorescent, especially if aging fluorescent tubes tend to flicker.

Modified lampshades. You can turn an old-fashioned lamp with an open-end lampshade into a light-diffusing model in several different ways. A new translucent shade coupled with a strong silvered-end bulb increases the amount and diffusion of the light.

If a new shade isn't practical, you can line the old one with aluminum foil or coat its inside with aluminum paint to increase light reflection and make a diffusing muff for the shade's end. Cut a piece of cheesecloth or thin white sheeting four inches greater in diameter than the shade's open end. Hem the outside edge and fit with an elastic band. If your lamp has a center post, you may need to cut a hole for it to pass through. Fancy or multiple light-bulb lamps can only be fitted with a muff by using a slightly more complex method: allow some extra fullness in cutting out the material. Make and hem a slit from the muff's outside edge to the center hole. Put the muff in place. Overlap the edges of the slit, and secure them in place with basting or snaps. With such a diffuser in place, you can use larger lightbulbs without causing harsh shadows or glare.

Lightbulbs. When lightbulbs fall within your line of vision or are so thinly screened that you can outline their contours, white-coated bulbs soften illumination somewhat.

Windowshades and curtains. Cream-colored windowshades or glass curtains scatter sunlight through the room, bouncing it back off of light-colored walls, ceilings and floors.

Light-reflecting surfaces. You can fill in eye-tiring shadows by bouncing light off the walls, ceiling and floor, but only if the light actually bounces instead of soaking in. Dark colors absorb as much as 95 per cent of the light which strikes them. Light walls, off-white ceilings, and pale floor-coverings bounce from 70 to 90 per cent back into the room, and help a great deal in supplying diffuse light.

If you can't change colors in a room, you may be able to add reflecting panels of pegboard or drapery. My daughter hung a piece of off-white pegboard on the wall in front of her desk, for instance. Two pin-up lamps on the pegboard give much better light than most study lamps, at much lower cost. Light-colored drapes or hangings may also serve in this way.

Decoration. Besides bouncing light back into the room to fill in shadows, light-hued walls, furniture and floors cut eye-fatiguing contrast by their own relative brightness. The amount of light reaching your eye from a given object equals the amount bounced back into the room from its surface rather than the amount which falls upon it. When your eyes simultaneously see a white page and a dark desk or floor covering, the excessive contrast tires your eyes even if light falls equally on both objects.

When reading or doing close eye work, you want the material at which you are looking to stand out from its background. Since brightness naturally draws your gaze, you can concentrate most easily if your work is the brightest thing in view. Ideally, then, the room should be decorated in hues light enough not to contrast unduly with well-lit work, but still dull enough that even patches of wall and floor which catch direct beams of sunlight do not command attention through excess brightness. One large office decorated especially for eye-easing has tan floor coverings, white ceilings, pale blue-green walls and light gray furnishings, for instance.

Cutting off your view to control contrast. Most people can't afford to decorate a room or office specifically to soothe their eyes and prevent excessive "brain" fatigue. But almost everyone can afford some furniture rearrangement and possibly some drapes or panels to make everything *within their range of vision when seated in a certain chair* fit the ideal brightness ratios. You can:

Turn the easy chair in which you do most of your reading toward a nearby corner. With fairly light-hued walls and a reading light that shines over your shoulder, everything in your range of vision will have eye-easing, fairly even brightness. The same light would not reach across the room to brighten dark-colored furniture and floors.

Block off your view of the rest of the room with a light-colored screen or hanging. Just a foot or so behind my typewriter stands an old hospital screen with unbleached muslin panels. The dark bookshelves behind it made unpleasant contrast with my well-lit work area, but now stays hidden from my view.

Push your desk against a wall, and hang a panel of off-white pegboard above it. Whether you use pin-up lamps on the pegboard or depend on overhead lights, this arrangement will make everything in your field of vision almost equally bright when you sit at your desk and face the wall.

Eliminating glare. Over-bright background areas create extra eye-wearying contrast with the areas around them, and make it harder to concentrate by drawing your eyes away from your work. Most modern office furniture takes this fact into account, with dull-surfaced desktops and non-glossy paint. Even home furniture usually boasts a velvety lacquered surface rather than a shiny varnished one nowadays. With older furniture, you can often cut glare without refinishing. A desktop blotter or cloth runner effectively dampens glare from a shiny varnished surface. Glass-front picture frames often look just as good with the glare-producing glass removed. As a last resort, you can often trace the light which bounces into your eyes back to its source and scatter it at that point with a windowshade, diffusing muff or altered lighting arrangement.

OTHER EYE EASERS

A great deal of eye-wearying effort comes from turning your eyes away from their natural straight-ahead gaze. The tiny muscles which move your eyes have more nerve connections from the brain than any other muscle in your body. Part of the nervousness, irritability, and fatigue which plagues deskworkers and executives at the end of the day comes from tension in these particular muscles—tension which you can almost always avoid with simple tonic measures.

Eye-refreshing hand pressure. If you've been reading this book for quite a while, here's a refresher you can try right now:

> Close both eyes and press the heels of your hands into your eye sockets so that they push your eyes gently back into your head. The proper degree of pressure usually makes your eyes "see gray"—instead of everything looking black, it will look a light grayish color. Often you will see a dark outline about the same size as the pages you have been reading, especially if background lighting is poor enough to make for excessive contrast. Continue the pressure for about thirty seconds, or until the afterimage fades (which may occur only after it goes through several color changes). Then gently relieve the pressure and go on reading.

Hand pressure has two favorable effects: It takes all tension off the eye-moving muscles, which run from the back of the eye socket to the eyeball and ordinarily must hold the eye in place. And it milks back into the circulation some of the eye's fluid, which builds up in pressure during prolonged eye use. By combatting these important sources of eye discomfort at the same time that you give your eyes a rest, you can avoid the fuzziness and fatigue that otherwise often plague you after prolonged paperwork or reading. Try hand pressure every fifteen minutes or so while using your eyes for close work or reading. You'll find it adds a lot to your comfort and staying power.

Eye exercises. If any other muscles which you need for work or play tire easily, your first thought is exercises to build them up. Why not use the same approach to weak eye muscles? Actually, seeing itself involves no fatigue. If tension-generating excess contrast has been eliminated, almost all eye fatigue comes from eye-moving muscles which you can easily strengthen through exercise. Several times a day, go through this routine:

> Hold a pencil point twelve to eighteen inches in front of your face and fix your eyes upon it. Keeping your head absolutely still, slowly move the pencil point as far up as your eyes can follow. Hold for five seconds. Move the pencil point as far to the right as your eyes can follow. Hold for five seconds. Move the pencil point as far down as your eyes can follow. Hold for five seconds. Move the pencil point as far to the left as your eyes can follow. Hold for five seconds. Repeat three times, closing your eyes for a few moments' rest between repetitions if necessary. Go through the entire routine four times a day.

If eye fatigue comes from eye muscle weakness, this exercise should distinctly improve your staying power at paperwork or reading in about three weeks. Thereafter, one set of eye exercises a day will maintain your newfound capacities.

Eye-resting position. Before you read the next paragraph, close your eyes, stretch, and settle yourself comfortably in your chair. Then open your eyes without deliberately looking toward this book.

* * *

Unless your eyes centered on this page automatically, you could probably decrease strain on your eye muscles by reading in a different position. Eyes straight ahead with book propped or held at a straight-on angle about fifteen inches from your face help you to concentrate, and to keep on concentrating without fagging out or feeling muddleheaded. Whether you're bucking for higher college grades, want bigger paychecks, or just enjoy reading into the night without growing weary, such an eye-rest position will give you real help. Combined with flat-footed, straight-spined bone-balance of the kind described on p. 138, it will also measurably increase your over-all bodily and mental efficiency.

Eye washes. After an hour or more of close work, your eyes often feel tired and drawn. Sometimes they begin to matter at the corners, or become red-rimmed and irritated. A two-minute eye wash usually stops all that, and refreshes your eyes for another spell of work. An inexpensive eye cup, obtainable at any drugstore, makes eyewashing both easy and neat. You can easily carry out the whole procedure in an office washroom without changing or protecting your clothes.

You probably have the ingredients for a good eye wash in your kitchen or medicine chest. Use distilled water to avoid the chlorine which most tap water contains. If you do not have distilled water available, let tap water stand in an open jar or bowl for 24 hours to let the chlorine escape. Mix one level teaspoonful of boric acid to one pint of water. If there is any trace of undissolved powder, let the solution stand until it settles out. Pour off the clear part to another vessel before use.

You can use ordinary baking powder instead of boric acid if you wish, but be especially careful to let any grit settle out. Your druggist carries both boric acid solution (already mixed) and baking soda powders for eyewash purposes (known technically as Sodium Bicarbonate powders, 2.4 GM., U.S.P.). If he knows that you want th material for eyewash, he will be sure that it is entirely free of grit. If you use the powders, mix each one with half a cup of warm water.

To use an eyewash, fill your eyecup about two-thirds of the way with whichever solution you choose. Look straight down and bring the rim of the cup into contact with your eye socket. Tip your head back, keeping the eye cup in close contact so that none of the solution spills. Open and close your eye several times inside the solution, then tip your head forward again, and remove the cup. Repeat several times with fresh solution.

CHAPTER ELEVEN'S MAIN EYE EASERS FOR LASTING MENTAL AND EMOTIONAL VIGOR

Simple eye easers usually let brainworkers keep at it longer and more efficiently without developing the irritability and fatigue of "brainweariness." *Softer* and *more even* light, which lessens eye-confusing contrast, gives more relief than brighter light on your work itself. In fact, if the background cannot be brightened to at least approach that of your work, *dimmer* subject lighting may relieve eyestrain. Brightness matching that from a bare 100 watt bulb at three to four feet works best for ordinary print. Bounced or scattered light fills in harsh shadows and eases eye-fatiguing contrast. Modern lamps and fixtures will do the trick, but so will less expensive measures like foil caps, backward-shining bulbs, modified lampshades, white lightbulbs, light-diffusing windowshades or curtains, and lighter paint or pegboard panels. Colors used in room decoration can cut eye-tiring contrast without going so far as to produce distracting highlights. Or you can get the same effect by turning your chair toward a well-lit corner, blocking off the rest of the room with a curtain or screen, or pushing your desk against a light-reflective wall. Glare-fighting measures also prove worthwhile.

Several other eye easers often prove helpful. *Hand pressure* rests eye muscles and lessens fluid pressure within the weary eyes. *Exercises* build eye-moving muscle strength. Eye-rest *positions* decrease strain, and proper *washes* often relieve eye fatigue.

CHAPTER TWELVE

Color,
the Great Soother
and Stimulator

One of my patients has been blind from birth, but still uses many references to color in his daily speech. To him, a vivacious, always-cheerful nurse is "the lady in red." A calm and tranquil afternoon is "azure," while he describes the day he endures surgery as "that burnt-orange cataclysm." His favorite vacation spot is "bathed in a cool green," even when the whole landscape is blanketed in snow. After you talk with this man, you can't help but notice how color affects your mood. You pause when your own lips form words like "blue mood," "bright moment," and "brown study" to thank God for your own color sense.

I think my patient deliberately uses color-words to make your contact with his affliction an uplifting one. But he also finds these words meaningful, and the meanings almost universal. Color *does* affect personality, and personality determines choice of color. Color *does* influence mood and heighten or decrease activity. Color *does* set the stage for gaiety or calm.

Several objective experiments show how profoundly color can affect each man or woman, and how much it influences the functions of both body and mind:

An obstetrician at Johns Hopkins had the different labor rooms painted in various hues. Women who endured travail in a green or blue room needed a great deal less medicine for relief of pain than those in a red room.

At the University of Iowa, another researcher found that infants, who have had little or no chance to acquire color

182

preferences, cried less in blue light than in red, and were more physically active in red light than blue.

At U.C.L.A., experiments proved that blood pressure, sweat gland activity, frequency of eyeblinks and certain types of brainwave are distinctly influenced by color.

Still more important effects occur quite regularly in the vast majority of subjects tested, but cannot be easily and directly measured. Blues and greens soothe anxiety, reds increase it. Blues and greens decrease self-assertion, reds make people more aggressive. Blues and greens encourage thought, reds provoke more action. For instance:

In a school with several sections in each grade, alternate rooms were painted in reds or maroons and in soft blues or greens. At midterm, the classes were rearranged so that pupils previously in red-hued rooms went into blue or green ones and *vice versa.* When in the red rooms, students required over twice as many trips to the principal's office for disciplinary purposes as when in the blue or green rooms.

A drab-walled government office redecorated in blue-green, with tan floors and gray-green office equipment. Production leaped up 5.5 per cent—an efficiency gain which would let you accomplish your quota of work in home or office in twenty less days each year.

A factory where *physical* rather than *mental* exertions were required was redecorated in pink. Workers stayed alert through the day with much less prodding from supervisors and suffered less fatigue. Surveys before and after showed the color change increased the number of workers who felt satisfaction with the job.

With less firm buttressing by fact and figure, experts also assert that certain other qualities of color in your surroundings help to perk you up, soothe your nerves, or help you to concentrate. Leading examples:

Contrast between dark and light or between clashing hues

seems either disturbing or exciting. Bold figures and glittering contrast in costumes and sets seem essential to an exciting musical number on the stage. On the other hand, yellow chalk on green blackboards (which also contrast less sharply with surrounding walls) seems to have helped classroom discipline.

Subdued background helps you to concentrate. The brightest areas in your field of vision constantly attract your attention. At your office or shop, that means bright light on your work. At home, it means treating your living room as background for the people inside.

Acquired tastes make some rooms seem cozy, others cramped —some spacious, others uncomfortably vast—some attractively feminine, others affectedly full of frills—some warmly masculine, others stiff and barren. Everyone will not agree on which is which, but everyone acknowledges that such matters are important.

HOW TO PUT COLOR TO WORK IN YOUR DAILY LIFE

Generally speaking, then, you can use reds and yellows, with bold figures and distinct contrast to *stimulate* your mind and body. These elements uplift your mood, cause exhilaration, improve strength and energy, increase alertness and incline you toward *vigorous* physical activity. They also increase sexual excitement and "party spirit."

On the other hand, greens and blues with subdued figures and muted contrast will *soothe* and *tranquilize* your mind and body, set to rest anxiousness and tension, and promote contemplative, conversational or creative capabilities. Such calming color influences also aid relaxation and sleep.

"Soothe" or "Stimulate" lists. Take a pencil right now, and divide a sheet of paper into two columns. Mark one "soothe" and the other "stimulate." List each of your daily or weekly activities under one heading or the other, according to which effect you think would help the most. Remember that "stimulate" refers mainly to the body—quiet companionship, conversation and solitary mind-pursuits like listening to music; reading and thinking flourish best under soothing circumstances. Record only items of which you feel instantly sure: activities which color can greatly promote stand foursquare in one group or the other, so you can simply omit from both lists any activity which you can't readily place. You'll still have a long list of personal and family activities which you can make more pleasant and effective through color influence.

Relocating activities. You can put color influence to work for you *right now* with no redecoration or special equipment by identifying the more stimulating and the more soothing areas in your home, shop or office and moving activities into the most suitable decor. Almost everybody needs stimulation at breakfast time, for instance. A bright room decorated with boldly figured wallpaper or drapery and leaning toward red, coral, yellow or pink will help you to wake up fast and shake off early morning blues. Maybe your kitchen or a sunny side porch provides just the environment you need, and still involves less work than carrying your meal into the dining area. On the other hand, both wage-earners and housewives grow tense and irritable by dinner time. Any children in the household become raucous and argumentative by day's end. A soothing atmosphere which encourages calm conversation suits your needs much better at the supper hour, and the shift to a quietly decorated dining room may prove well worth the effort.

To take another example, my teenage daughter decided to take exercises every day, mainly to improve her figure. The most convenient room for this use happens to be decorated in soft tans and browns, and she found her enthusiasm lagging. A shift to our brightly-decorated kitchen (at bedtime when the room isn't otherwise in use) made the exercises seem much easier and more invigorating.

You'll find that many of the activities on your "soothe" and "stimulate" lists can simply be moved to a suitable spot. Perhaps you can merely change the direction in which you face, or put the room's blinds up or down: in my own home, we usually eat on a breezeway-porch, but adjust the basswood shades to flood the room with sunshine and open out the view for "perk-up" breakfasts or to bounce the light around the green-painted room and close us into a cozy space for calmer evening meals.

Colored lights. Often you can create an appropriate atmosphere by different lighting for an activity which you cannot move. Your house may provide only one suitable place for dining— a room decorated in soft greens or blues for tranquil family living. But when you stow the kids in bed and celebrate your anniversary with a midnight supper, dim candlelight gives the whole room a seductive red-yellow tone. When you invite your friends in for a gay party, hidden red floodlights of the kind sold to shine on silvered Christmas trees bounce exciting highlights off one wall to set a party mood.

You can use drapes or blinds to change room light, too. Half-translucent blinds can mute the colors in almost any room. Thin blue or greenish draperies in a matching room tint the walls a deeper hue when drawn across the entering sunlight, and turn a moderately soothing atmosphere into an intensely soothing one. In a red-hued room, dimmed reddish light from drawn draperies lacks the brightness needed to spur intensive physical exertion. Generally speaking, the brighter light of open drapes and freely-admitted sunlight helps you to get through your housework more easily than dim reddish light (although bright reddish or yellowish light would be ideal).

Different colored lights in central fixtures and floor lamps may also fit into your plans. One of my wealthier friends decorated his living room in whites and grays, then installed three different lighting circuits, one white, one rose and one soft blue. The rose light is both complimentary and stimulating, adding distinctly to the gaiety of parties and get-togethers. The blue soothes his mood during solitary reading or resting periods after a tension-wracked day. The white makes the room look crisp and cool on a summer night, and serves for most family occasions. You can accomplish the same ends with a few colored lightbulbs if you wish. White light from central fixtures and reading lamps give basic light. A blue-bowled lamp or blue lightbulb in a TV lamp will soothe you during periods of solitude, when other lamps can be turned off. Its light should be quite dim, so only a single bulb is probably needed. Whether you're thinking through a problem, listening to music or just relaxing, you'll find blue light helpful for inward-turned pursuits. Red-colored floodlights concealed so that they bounce off an unbroken wall or against drawn drapes will bounce their exciting light back into the room, either to add stimulation while the white lights still burn or to create a sex-ually stimulating glow with other lamps turned off.

You might also consider putting rose-hued lightbulbs of the type sold as sources of complimentary soft light into at least one set of bedroom lamps. Their reddish hue may prove mildly stim-ulating sexually, and often helps you to wake up a bit more quickly in the morning.

Redecorating for the sake of color effects. You don't need to spend much money on redecoration to benefit enor-mously from color effects. The areas where color can do you the most good are the least expensive to redecorate. Just remember that physical tasks go faster and seem easier in brightly lit rooms painted yellow, peach or pink, possibly with a few boldly colored decorations. Thinking-reading-listening-talking activities of or-dinary family living go much better in softer light and cooler hues—gray, blue, green or turquoise—with subdued decoration and muted contrast. For study and paperwork, use the same col-ors, but brighten the room sufficiently to avoid any eyestrain. Check each area against this list:

Your laundry area. Basement laundries usually are gloomy, drab and depressing. A few panels of coral-painted pegboard or even an old set of pastel-hued drapes to conceal the dark, bare studs may work wonders. Add brighter and rosier lighting—perhaps a couple of goosenecked pin-up lamps with their light bounced off the pegboard—to make laundry-day chores easier to bear.

Workshop. Household repairs and odd jobs deserve a work center at home. Such jobs get done sooner, faster and easier when the workbench is convenient, pleasantly decorated, and well lit. Coral, yellow or pink-painted pegboard with pin-up lamps directed against it gives an ideal energizing backdrop. A gallery of bright pictures or cartoons doesn't hurt. In my own basement, I've stapled building paper printed with a ceiling design (obtained from Montgomery Ward for a few cents a roll) to the bottom of the joists, which seals off dust, dampens spread of noise, and makes the whole area brighter and more pleasant.

Kitchen. Brightness everywhere and bold figure in the small areas left between appliances and cabinets helps to make this center of housewife's workday a positive aid to getting the job finished. Most of the work is mainly physical, so yellows, corals, pinks or reds deserve emphasis in decorating. Sharp contrast with bright green or blue figures may also fit in, so long as the stimulating colors predominate.

Perhaps working wives and live-alone bachelors might find the accumulated tensions of the working day aggravated by such an environment. I've noticed that such people—and an occasional child-harried housewife—seem to like a quieter kitchen. Judge your own needs, but decorate to suit them.

Breakfast room. Since most people need to be stimulated at breakfast time and soothed at supper, a separate eating area for the morning meal usually proves worthwhile. Its color needs conform with those of the kitchen, which often proves an ideal breakfast spot. If you have space for a separate breakfast nook, keep its decoration sprightly.

Dining area. Soft greens or blues please! Harried housewives and weary workers need to be soothed, and children are always fractious by this time of day.

Living room and recreation area. Even when the members of our family greatly outnumbered the number of rooms in the house, we always have set up a separate "rumpus room" or basement play zone. Living rooms should be decorated for quiet conversation and companionship, while most families need a place for raucous get-togethers, too. This is especially true when the children are young, but when they get older you've got the grandchildren to think about—and what grandparent doesn't want to entice the wee ones to his house somehow?

Bedrooms. In most households, bedrooms are centers of privacy and therefore of solitary pursuits. Blues and greens prove most suitable for such activities. The first stirrings of sex interest, in which color makes the biggest difference, usually take place elsewhere, so few couples need a sexually stimulating color environment.

Office or plant. You probably can't control decoration and lighting in your work place very well, but if possible suit these conditions to your personal needs.

Colored glasses. When you cannot choose the color of your surroundings, you can still control the color of light reaching your eyes. Although researchers find that colored light shining on your skin measurably affects your pulse and breathing, most action probably comes through effect upon your eyes. Bluish or blue-green lenses often help to soothe undue tensions, whether or not eyestrain has any part in their causation. Rose-tinted lenses sometimes perk you up during mild depression and do-nothing spells.

Avoiding color overdose effects. One caution in the use of color: you must seek surroundings which *harmonize with* rather than *counteract* your more extreme moods. When very depressed, as during a period of mourning, gay surroundings seem inept rather than cheering. Extreme anxiety or excitement has the opposite effect, making a calm environment seem upsetting. Use color action to give you a little boost rather than a kick in the pants, and a mild soothing effect instead of an anesthetic. Within its limitations, color influence can add tremendous zest and mellowness to your life, but you'll only become discouraged if you use it against overwhelming odds.

CHAPTER TWELVE'S MAIN POINTS ON COLOR AS A TONIC AND REFRESHER

Color affects both mind and body in many measurable ways. Reds and yellows, perhaps with blocks of contrasting blues and shades, excite and stimulate you. They can help you get a quick start in the morning, work faster on physical tasks, and stir excitement at parties or in sexual preliminaries. Greens and blues, perhaps with subdued light and muted contrast, soothe your tensions, quiet tempers, and promote thought instead of action. They can help you toward more peaceful dinnertime conversation, quiet your jangled nerves, and aid you in thinking through your problems.

You can put color to work for you by listing activities and occasions which either soothing action or stimulation would help. In many cases, a simple change of scene will do the trick. You can move each activity to a suitably decorated part of your house. In other cases, colored light may give the answer: either colored light bulbs or natural light filtered through colored drapes or shades. You may also find redecoration worthwhile, especially in areas like the basement laundry and workshop. Wake-up breakfasts call for different color influence than end-of-a-hard-day suppers, and recreation periods have different requirements than companionable evenings. Colored glasses extend color influence to areas whose lighting and decoration you do not control. However, you can't fight strong emotions with color: you're more comfortable in an atmosphere which harmonizes with them.

CHAPTER **THIRTEEN**

Aesthetic Lifts
and Bracers

Primitive mood-boosters 194, Developed appreciations 200, Summary 202.

Americans usually seek recreation with impact instead of subtle uplift. Yet gentle pleasures offer unique aid when you feel weary or tension-ridden. They occupy your mind, restore your mood, and simultaneously help you to relax instead of imposing their own burdens of fatigue or undue excitement.

PRIMITIVE MOOD-BOOSTERS

When the Three Kings brought the Infant Jesus gold, frankincense and myrrh, they proved that they were Wise Men indeed. For here were gifts even an infant could appreciate—gifts pleasing to sight, smell and taste without need for training in appreciation.

Today, lifts and bracers which require no acquired taste are no longer rarities for the royal few. You can bathe yourself in beautiful colors, scent the air with compounds rare or nonexistent in the past, and enjoy flavors which no Asian potentate of any former age could savor.

Natural beauty. Most new homes have a picture window. The "picture" may include a dirty street and the neighbor's cluttered driveway, but it also embraces green grass, blue sky and perhaps a few attractive bushes or flowers. Each glimpse of these things may prove a sort of tonic. You get a boost over and over again as you glance at landscape, or look out over the city from a pleasantly situated office.

If you can't look out at natural beauty, maybe you can introduce some into your own living room. For instance:

House plants take very little care, and may give you a soothed and refreshed feeling every time your gaze rests upon them. Proper selection depends mainly on available space and light. In a basement apartment, you can light a desk or table with a wall-hung fluorescent fixture, sold at low cost in the mail order catalogues for use above a stove. African violets will grow profusely on small shelves and brackets beneath the fixture as well as on the back of the table. Upstairs, a little natural sunlight supports a lot of philodendron greenery. More direct light with little space might make a cactus garden best, while both light *and* space opens a wide range of possibilities for flowering and decorative plants.

A dancing *fire* in a fireplace fights boredom and boosts mood without interfering with thought or conversation. Here in Minnesota, birchwood and hickory fires are favorites—the former because its beautiful bark contrasts with the licking flames, the latter because of its power to scent the air. Cannel coal or even artificial fires have a hearty beauty too. Rugged masculine types usually enjoy a fire more than any other type of decoration, and companionability seems to flourish under its influence.

Birds or other house pets can add color and interest, as well as companionship. You can keep parrots and parakeets without any appreciable health risks, since the disease they spread to humans yields readily to new medicines and is very rare. Canaries almost never carry any germs capable of attacking humans. Some dogs and cats display constant grace and beauty.

Other people. You don't gather friends and family for their beauty as you collect decorative cups, but too often you almost forget to nurture their attractiveness. Remember the old saying: "Behind every great man there's a good woman." Certainly, a good woman creates a setting in which her husband and family flourish—a home which subtly cheers and spurs them on when they require such push, and quiets or soothes them when they need a rest. But there is a deeper wisdom in this piece of folk wisdom: a recognition of the aesthetic lift and mood-sustained beauty which one person certainly can offer to another. Not fleshly beauty, or at least not that alone. The sum of all the things that make a husband feel more confidence and cheer when his wife is sitting across the living room, or make a wife feel proud and grateful when her family gathers around—these are the human lifts and bracers with which each household should abound, which each of us can work hard to provide for our own family, and which deserve appreciation.

Or take children. I know of few parents who never feel a thrill from catching their youngsters in a certain pose or in a certain light. But I know a great many who miss nine-tenths of such uplift simply by failing to look. For such a parent, the best prescription may be a camera. You can train yourself to see beauty and interest, and one of the best ways to do so is to look for moments worth preserving with film. In many cases, the need to write letters about your children also helps. When you write to Grandma once a week, you remain constantly alert for incidents which bear repeating. Perhaps if you have not enjoyed your children's attractions several times daily, you should keep a diary for a few weeks, to train yourself in perceiving their intriguing moments.

Of course, human beauty can be enhanced. Not long ago, my wife hung a full length mirror in the hallway, mainly to aid her seamstresship (since she makes her own clothes). To get from the bedroom to the breakfast table, the whole family had to walk past that mirror. Almost all of us—including myself—suffered some shock at seeing how we looked. Perhaps part of our breakfast grumpiness was simply a response to the disheveled view! Not a word was said about better grooming, but we found a great deal more combed hair and brushed teeth around us as we glanced around the table.

Such simple things can add considerable uplift to family life. Of course, no one can keep small children completely neat all day, but a little effort, gradual training, and a good example can make a big difference to your household atmosphere.

Incense and perfume. When I was in medical school, one of my teachers claimed that cigarette smoke has almost no taste, and that most smokers could only tell that their cigarette was lit through their senses of vision and smell. A group of my classmates tested this statement. Each member of the group in turn was blindfolded. While other fellows blew smoke in his face to neutralize his sense of smell, he puffed on an unlit or on a lit cigarette. Only two out of ten consistently could tell which was which.

With millions of Americans surrendering years of their lifespan for a pleasure whose main element is scent, it seems ironic that our nation frowns on incense. Here is a harmless, inexpensive, unobtrusive mood-booster acclaimed by millions of people in other parts of the world. Yet because our books and plays link it with pagan rites, with dark mysterious Orientals or other unpleasant things, very few of us take advantage of its benefits.

These benefits are fundamentally three: first, incense is pleasant and mood-boosting, but completely unobtrusive. You can enjoy its pleasures in some nook or cranny of your brain without decreasing your concentration on other pursuits. You can work or read, converse or make love with pleasant odors wafting gently about, and not divert attention from its target. Second, no other sense affects your emotions as directly and immediately as sense of smell. In dealing with mood—the keystone of vigor and of satisfaction with life—the sense of smell has an inside track. Third, odors quickly become linked in your mind with emotions, attitudes and values. A scent which lingers through an episode of loving intimacy will subtly renew affection and sexual excitement on similar occasons. In the same way, an odor linked to camaraderie will soon enhance the pleasant effects of a companionable evening, and an odor associated with relaxed solitude will soon prove quieting in its own right.

You can use incense either as a natural refresher or as a mood-setting tonic for relaxation, companionship or affection. The cost is slight, the equipment simple, the time spent almost none. As each incense-burning recalls the emotional atmosphere of previous occasions, its mood-building action will steadily increase. Of course, perfume and scented toilet aids can be used similarly. However, they tend to be associated more with the *person* than with the *occasion* and do more to influence relationships than moods.

Long-lasting flavor. Along with nicotine, tar, and spittoon-hitting ammunition, a quid of chewing tobacco feeds a steady stream of strong flavor into your mouth. Old-timers find the constant, pungent taste very stimulating indeed.

Chances are you wouldn't put up with chewing-tobacco mess no matter how lively the habit made you feel. However, other long-lasting flavors can perk you up or keep you refreshed as time wears on. Chewing gum and sucking candies make good lasting-flavor energizers, but with unfortunate effects on cavity formation and weight control. A number of highly-flavored preparations work equally well without these drawbacks, such as:

Sugarless chewing gum, diabetic hard candy, noncaloric fruit-flavored punches made from special powder, all on sale at drug and grocery stores.

Homemade popsicles or snowballs made from noncaloric punches or with lemon juice and Sucaryl liquid.

Lemonade with lots of chopped ice, made with Sucaryl rather than sugar and either fresh or bottled lemon juice, and sipped slowly.

Cloves or other spices chewed or sucked.

Sounds. If you've ever awakened out in the woods, whether in camp or cottage, you know how the rustle of breeze-stirred leaves and the twittering song of birds starts the day right. You listen, you smile, you stretch—how much more refreshing than rolling out to the sound of an alarm clock! Through the rest of the day, gentle woods sounds continually cheer and invigorate you.

You can enjoy similarly pleasant sounds in your own home or office. Glass chimes tinkling together in the gentle breeze or in the airstream from a heating duct brighten the deadly quiet of a lonely house. Canaries and parakeets chirp pleasantly. Chiming or cuckoo clocks add a touch of cheerful interest to your day without obtruding on your consciousness. Even the steady tick of a pendulum-type clock can prove very soothing: one of my psychiatrist friends found that a clock ticking about once each second definitely relieved the tension which long silences otherwise created during interviews with his patients. Both housewives and executives might benefit from this discovery.

Textures. All of my children have been very attached to a certain blanket in their infancy. They have clutched it when they needed solace, and stroked it as they went to sleep. Sometimes only a few tattered strips remained before they were ready to give up the familiar-feeling comforter—the intimate, immediate reminder of past love and quiet.

Emotional associatons may explain texture's effects. Or perhaps more primitive responses are involved, since textures that resemble soft skin seem to have special appeal. At any rate, most people get a subtle uplift from touching a piece of well-tanned leather, from sliding between smooth, crisp sheets, or from the soft caress of whisper-soft negligee. Most men enjoy texture mainly in things they hold in their hands, while women get uplift from textures which touch any part of their bodies. In either case, a gift with a beautiful feel will give pleasure and uplift quite often. Why not obtain such things often for your family—and for yourself?

DEVELOPED APPRECIATIONS

When my wife and I moved to Minneapolis, we found the city a well-developed center for modern art.

"Maybe we're missing something," my wife said. So we enrolled in a night school class in art appreciation. Neither of us became a fanatic—we still don't own a single painting or piece of sculpture. But a painting which we wouldn't previously have *tried* to appreciate sometimes now gives one or the other of us a moving, soothing or invigorating experience.

You can learn to appreciate a great many things that you would never enjoy spontaneously. A great many of life's pleasures depend on learning, or at least on willingness to try new things. As one of my art class friends remarked: "If nobody developed new tastes, there would be an awful shortage of mothers' milk."

Perhaps most new tastes grow from experiences you get without making an effort—meals you eat because your parents serve them, music you hear because the radio keeps you from feeling lonely and bored. But everyone in the world can get enjoyment and satisfaction from *something* which he has not yet discovered or learned to appreciate. Developing such interests makes you feel more intellectually vigorous, more cheerful, more lively—more all-around *youthful*—than you'll feel if you stick to old pleasures.

Art doesn't have to be "deep" or expensive to perk up your mood and revive your vigor. One of my mechanic patients "recharges his batteries" by running his eye along a pin-up gallery that is anything but obscure. Another friend collects inexpensive reproductions of famous paintings, "rotates the crop" on his walls once a month. Nor is it necessary to show off your treasures to enjoy them. A lawyer friend of mine keeps his one expensive painting in a back room where clients seldom go. "That's where

I do my reading and research," he told me. "Whenever my brain starts to feel fuzzy, a few moments of communing with that picture livens me up again."

Almost everyone can surround himself for at least part of the day with things he loves to see or touch. If you start looking for the art objects which mean the most to you when used in this way, you might wind up with anything from model airplanes to a Picasso pot. Whatever turn your interests take, you'll probably achieve something worthwhile. Your newly-developed tastes will add islands of refreshment and invigorating lift to your days throughout succeeding years, often at negligible cost.

Music not only has powers to calm the madding beast, but does pretty well with ordinary, everyday tensions. If worries run around in your head and keep you from relaxing when you lie down during the day, try resting to music—classical, semiclassical, popular lyrics or low-key jazz. Put on a favorite record, lie down and follow the relaxing routine on p. 82. Or play music softly in the background to set the mood for a pleasant mealtime conversation or quiet family evening.

Music can be stimulating, too. Well-chosen numbers can put you in the mood for everything from a gay party to an exchange of marital intimacies, can help you to wake up in the morning or revive yourself after a tough day's work.

Your own tastes govern what kind of music works best for you, but it never hurts to sample all types available before you settle into a groove. You might be surprised at what you like best, after a broad sampling.

One unusual use for music: to make people "speak up" so that oldsters can hear them. The dulled hearing which afflicts so many people in their sixties, seventies and eighties usually causes trouble with soft voices. When people adjust their voices to overcome background music, the oldsters can hear much better than in a dead-quiet room.

Article design can boost your spirits, too. Most people think of

appreciation only in terms of works intended solely to communi-
cate ideas or feelings—poetry, art, music and the like. But a
beautiful building, a well-designed chair, a lovely dress or an
attractive vase can also give you a lift. Although such things serve
other purposes, they also affect your mood. Pick them to live with
as well as to serve their purposes, and everything from clothes to
kitchen utensils will add moments of soothing appreciation to
your life.

Mementos. In the hundreds of home visits I've made to
patients, I've noticed one thing: men and women who move
through their sixties and seventies with contentment and satisfaction almost always have a room full of mementos, while a
barren room often goes with a barren life. Of course, a life that
leads to a roomful of mementos may produce happier senior
years. But I firmly believe that part of the difference comes from
the mementos themselves—that when you have a great deal of
living to look back across, reminders of its high spots give real
and continual boosts.

If you're still in your building years, gather mementos to
brighten your future. Take family portraits, save souvenirs from
every graduation, wedding, christening or big event, collect
souvenirs of trips and visits. Remember that you'll benefit more
from items you can keep constantly in view or available than
from items that wind up in the attic. Photos you can frame and
display benefit you more than ones you put into an album, while
you'll see more of pictures in an album than of dried roses or
bright-colored coral that clashes with the rest of your decor.

If you have built your life already, set out your souvenirs.
Good moments, like good friends, deserve to be revisited quite
often.

AESTHETIC LIFTS AND BRACERS REVIEWED

You don't need artificial "culture" to get a boost from many
aesthetic lifts and bracers. *Natural beauty* from the view through

your windows to house plants, a cozy fire or a caged bird may give a lift. The other *people* in your household may have attractions, too, if you train yourself to look for them. *Incense* quickly acquires emotional values through which you can relax, set the mood for companionship or affection, and enhance the emotional value of various experiences. *Long-lasting or piquant flavors* perk you up to some degree, and need not involve bad effects on teeth or waistline. Sugarless sweets, homemade noncaloric ices and ades, or chewed spices work very well. Pleasant *sounds* add touches of cheer or soothing effect.

Like skills, appreciations can be learned. Give yourself a chance to experience the soothing or invigorating effects which can come to you through *art, music* and *design*. Gather and display *mementos,* search out the inward beauty of the human beings with whom you share your days.

Life's little pleasures keep you cheerful, alert and interested in what goes on around you—advantages without which you would accomplish very little. Pleasure for its own sake seems almost immoral to some people, but pleasure for the sake of new efficiency and enhanced vigor makes sense even to Puritans. Perhaps this chapter will lead you toward many new sources of such stimulation.

CHAPTER FOURTEEN

Mind Tonics:
Diversions, Recreations
and Emotional
Safety Valves

You can paddle a thousand miles through primitive lakes and streams near Ely, Minnesota. One or two portages back, the fish bite as if they've never seen a lure (which most of them haven't). Blue water and green forest stretch as far as the eye can see. Days might pass before your party comes in hailing distance of another. The cares of civilization quickly wash away in the cold, clear water and the crisp, clean air, leaving you physically fit, mentally alert, and emotionally rejuvenated.

Maybe "roughing it" in the woods doesn't appeal to you. But almost anything you choose to revive your interest in life and rejuvenate your outlook *differs* from what you ordinarily do, and *captivates* your interest. Let's see what you can do *right now,* without taking an expensive trip or losing a lot of time from work, to accomplish those mind-refreshing ends.

DESKSIDE OR STAY-AT-HOME DIVERSIONS

When you come up against the same blank wall over and over again in your thinking, it often helps to lay the matter aside for a few days. When you come back to it "fresh," the answer you previously couldn't reach may instantly pop into your head. But what if you can't seem to shake off a problem so that you can come back to it fresh? What if you keep worrying and worrying without getting anywhere? Or what if you just can't take time to "sleep on" a big decision?

A captivating *diversion* breaks the self-defeating pattern. It lets you come back to your problem mentally refreshed and ready to see new and different approaches.

Creative diversions often work best. You can throw yourself into a creative project completely, adjusting its scope to continually "stretch" your talent. The emotional frustrations which accompany an unsolved problem, an unresolved worry, or a troublesome relationship often find relief in creative expression, too. I've seen anger and fear splashed raw upon paper with finger paints: great slashes of vivid color applied with a grimacing face and clawed hands—and followed by the serenity of a blown-out storm.

Although many famous men, like Winston Churchill, have found release and mind refreshment in oil paints or water colors, media much easier to master let you blow off steam and serve as suitable distractions. You may find satisfaction in finger paints, pastels, charcoal drawing or pencil sketches. Modeling in clay, soap carving or simple whittling take up little space and need not make much mess. Wood carving in relief, engraving, etching, copperwork and other varieties of artistic craft can be done in whole or part out of a desk drawer as well as in a shop. A few of my patients have set up more complex affairs—a potter's wheel, stone-carving equipment, and so on.

Less creative *crafts* can occupy your mind completely, even though they give less outlet for emotional constraint. Some can be done at deskside, like tying flies or making jewelry. Others require special equipment and space, like dressmaking and woodwork. But if you take on tasks which call for all your skill, any craft gets you "away from it all" completely.

A variety of PUZZLES and ARTIFICIAL PROBLEMS also distract a worried mind. Among the popular choices:

Crossword puzzles and similar word games.

"How would you play this hand" self-quizzes based on newspaper or magazine columns giving bridge hands, autobridge self-played hands, self-dealt cards.

Solitaire. Several books explain numerous varieties.

Problems in chess or checkers. A folding board and book or magazine page fits into any desk drawer.

Packaged problem boards such as Hoo-Doo and Bewitched.

Pets also provide apt distraction. Even in a busy office, you can keep an ant colony or a bowl of tropical fish. Dogs provide fond intervals of mood-restoring play, while songbirds and parakeets provide different forms of pleasant companionship.

Perhaps the simplest diversions are mere TRICKS OF MIND. Whenever one doctor friend of mine finds himself stumped by a patient's illness, he leans back in his chair, closes his eyes, and does two or three problems of long division in his head. When he gets back to the case at hand, his fresh view of the case often reveals an answer. One of my patients used a similar trick to banish paralyzing worries about his sexual strength. For years, the least shred of doubt made him concentrate upon his incapacity. Attempts to think of sexually stimulating things only made matters worse—the more he tried to conjure up erotic visions, the less excitement he would feel. But when he tried to multiply three-figure numbers together in his head, all other thoughts and worries disappeared. Instead of building impulse-wrecking spirals of fear, his mind became serenely blank and his body ready for response.

Finally, you may find some need for chink-filling distractions —tasks to fill up the unused corners of your intellect when your major activities fail to occupy your full attention. A lagging conversation, dull TV program or mechanical task leaves part of your mind free to wander. Your intellect then settles upon worries or trains of thought which interfere with what you are doing. Knitting, drawing pictures on a scratch pad, darning socks or any of the dozens of semi-automatic tasks may actually help to keep your mind *on* a halfway-occupying activity by keeping it *off* more completely distracting concerns.

EMOTIONAL OUTLETS

One of my farmer patients used to vent his spleen on the woodlot. For years after he could have afforded a chain saw, he chopped his way through log after log, being notably more vigorous in his swings just after an argument with his wife.

A white-haired colonel's wife told me her favorite outlet—the Irish technique of scrubbing the kitchen floor. Hair in a loose bun, shapeless and overlarge dress, kneeling pad and stiff-bristled brushes all formed part of a ritual which left her tired but relaxed and free from accumulated pique.

A mild-mannered young bank clerk went with me to a nearby driving range and walloped his first shot 250 yards.

"You really laid into that ball," I remarked.

Smiling sweetly, he replied:

"First time I've really let go all day."

Each of these people had found by experience that violent action eased certain types of turmoil and emotional upset. You can gain the same type of release, and perhaps make it more effective, if you recognize this fact:

Violent emotions dissipate themselves in violent physical acts, even if those acts strike out at a target which has nothing to do with the original upset.

You can unload burdens of pent-up anger and quench the smoldering coals of hatred—nasty emotions which darken your mood and hamper your relationships with friends and family— with pleasant or useful activities of properly chosen sorts. You don't even have to admit to yourself or others that such feelings exist (which may prove hard in a society which has trained you from birth to maintain a spirit of friendly cooperation). Any sport, hobby or task involving violent assault against an object or animal gives hostility-release type refreshment. Hunting and

fishing are Minnesota favorites. Darts and archery give good release, especially if you use balloons or other destructible objects
as targets. Crafts involving sawing, pounding, chipping or cutting relieve pent-up turmoil. Even watching violence may help:
you can feel sufficiently involved with your favorite boxer,
wrestler or football team to feel exhilarating release from crunch-
ing blows and charges.

Antidotes for a "slow burn." Persistent anger, resentment
or hostility casts a pall upon your own life and that of those who
live with you. When you know exactly what is "eating you" and
exactly who is at fault, you can use a more specific antidote instead of a general emotional outlet. Voodoo practitioners make
a wax doll to resemble the offender, then stick pins through it or
beat it with sticks. I rather doubt that this treatment actually
makes the offender sick, but it certainly makes the voodoo priest's
onlooking customer feel better. Pinning an offender's picture to
the target at which you shoot darts, arrows or bullets also gives
real and immediate release. Merely thinking of the boss's slope-
shouldered figure as you take aim at a bowling pin will make the
sport more satisfying, and a golfer can add twenty yards to each
drive if he thinks of his mother-in-law's head. Similar revenge-
fantasy fits into most violent games and activities—you can think
of your wife's leg as you chop logs or of your boss's bland face
when you clout a volleyball.

You might think that such thoughts of violence would lead to
lost self-control and make you a potential Lizzie Borden. Nothing could be farther from the truth. You'll find your pent-up
anger easily forgotten, and thoughts of harsh revenge with them,
after you've blown off steam. Self-control and civilized behavior
become much easier when you have an acceptable outlet. And
these outlets *are* acceptable, both because everybody uses them
and because the expressions of hostility they permit remain completely secret. Nobody need ever know what you are thinking to
make your release do its work.

Airing grievances and disturbance. "If I had my life to live over——."

How often have you heard that heart-rending phrase? Next time one of your friends or family uses it, interrupt by saying:

"Live your life again, *right now.*"

You *can* relive your life to some extent—at least the episodes from which emotional residues still rankle. You can get a second chance to express regret about events you didn't want to happen, or to make a sharp retort to an unwarranted insult. You can recreate events, at least so far as their emotional significance is concerned, by talking about what you did, and how you felt, and what you wish you'd done instead. You relive the past in your mind's eye through conversation, and to some extent set it emotionally straight.

Suppose you tell your wife:

"The boss had no business bawling me out. I pushed the right buttons, but the blasted machine didn't work. I should have told him off, that's what I should have done. None of it was *my* fault!"

Your wife will probably agree with you. But her reassurance doesn't really matter: it's the airing of your grievance that makes the difference. You feel better when you've expressed what you now feel you should have said or done, even if you couldn't possibly have taken such a course of action. The same holds true of episodes which leave you feeling guilty or doubtful about your own behavior.

Friends and *family* make good confidants for relatively minor, day-to-day disturbances. Your husband or wife will gladly listen to your experiences at work or with the children, your friends at work will gladly discuss problems on the home front, and all of them will gladly discuss each other. With rare exceptions, though, you can't blow off about big issues to your family or friends. Your pride and your need for standing with these people won't let you dwell continually on your involvement in dubious episodes, even if you can be sure your confidences will be kept. You must always think about the future of your personal relationships, and keep from discussing issues which will later make you embarrassed in your confidant's company.

For really big issues, the best confidant may be a "professional." Most rabbis, ministers and priests listen sympathetically and keep confidences completely. Social workers in Family Service agencies (which often function on an ability-to-pay basis for everyone, not for charity clients alone) will lend a compassionate ear. Marriage counselors, family doctors, clinical psychologists and psychiatrists listen much more than they talk. All of these "good listeners" usually prove much more helpful and much less expensive in the long run than bartenders or chance acquaintances, who deserve mention only because of their great popularity for this role.

For "in between" upheaval—too deep-rooted to discuss with friends but not so vital as to justify professional consideration— other outlets often yield emotional peace and mental refreshment. You can review events in *prayer*, which often gives absolution for your guilts and helps you to accept with tranquility the offenses which have bred anger. You can write vituperative or confessing *letters*, which you will probably tear up or burn once the free expression of your feelings has relieved their urgency. You can express your feelings in a *creative work* of music or art—a fingerpainting, a bit of molded clay, a poem, story or play. The characters and episodes need not stand out in recognizable form to make self-expression a tonic to guilt-weary or resentful souls. Rankling emotion cries for self-expression, and pours out through any channel you may supply.

FRIENDSHIP AND LOVE

Sharing beneficial emotions with a friend or loved one gives extra pleasure. Sharing hurtful emotions gives real relief. These effects make friendship and love the greatest mind-tonics of all.

Potential **sharing of emotion as a mind-tonic and support.** If you know that someone else would keenly respond to your sorrows if he knew about them, you feel solace and support. Even if the other person is far away and cannot possibly know anything about your troubles, the fact that he would be concerned if he knew means a great deal to you.

Potential sharing rather than *actual* determines the depth of friendship or love. The bridegroom who scans the newspaper before rushing off to work neither wants nor welcomes his bride's passionate approach, but he measures his love by the sharing they can achieve when the time is ripe, not by its failure to click at inept moments.

To a large extent, open pathways for emotion also have more to do with the tonic effects of companionship than the use that is made of them. The husband who reads a detective thriller while his wife mends socks across the room may not share his feelings, but still enjoys her presence. *Potential* sharing builds with each peak of *actual emotional sharing* you experience. Sharing the *experiences* directly or through later conversation helps only if you share emotions, too.

Open-heartedness and friendship or love. The extent to which you let others in on your feelings and the extent to which you respond to theirs makes a tremendous difference. Excessive reserve blocks broadcast of feeling, disinterest or intellectualization prevents reception of it. Either serves as a wet blanket on the development of closer friendships and loves.

Most of us are afraid to wear our hearts on our shirtsleeves. When people know *all* your feelings, they have tremendous power to hurt you. Moreover, we don't respect "gushers" who express exaggerated feeling about each and every issue, so we lean over backwards to avoid this fault. However, several concrete steps will safely spread your feelings to others and safely increase your awareness of theirs in a way which almost always makes for closer friendship and deeper bonds of affection.

1. Seek "shared-feeling" experiences. Some activities give more opportunities for shared feeling than others. Consider the difference between dancing together, where you pay close attention to every nuance of your partner's movement, and watching TV, where the *program* rather than the *other person* gets your main attention. Sports and games, trips or excursions, partnership projects, and agreeable conversation usually involve the most easily-arranged types of togetherness, suitable for friends or family alike, in which shared emotion is almost automatic.

2. Let most emotions flow forth unrestrained. Youngsters need emotional reserve or camouflage, because they haven't learned which feelings are "safe"—which ones they can reveal without offending others or losing stature. Later in life, you rarely need to delay expression of emotion for censorship. You can express yourself much more freely with most people and in most circumstances. You generally make yourself more likable and lovable (as well as less constrained) in the process.

Probably you can best attack the habit of emotional constraint first in your own home or with your closest friends, where an occasional goof won't wreck your relationships. Don't try to express emotion in words: just let your feelings flow freely in gesture, facial expression, tone of voice, and so forth. If you feel like putting your hand on your son's shoulder, don't worry about whether it will make you seem too sentimental. If a news story on TV touches your heart, say "Isn't that too bad?" in the sorrowful tone that comes natural instead of shuddering to yourself. A close call in traffic might call for "Whew—that was a close one" instead of grin-and-bear-it self-restraint. Naturally you don't want to express feelings which will hurt people, or those of which you'll later feel ashamed—but a lifetime of refinement has made both varieties much rarer than you might suppose.

After you let down your hair deliberately with your family and best friends for a few weeks, stop and take stock. Have you drawn your friends closer by making them more aware of the "real you" or driven them away by revealing too much? Have you refreshed your brain by airing many feelings which would otherwise have rankled, or imposed new feelings of guilt upon it through social blunders? Have you enjoyed your experiences more through expression-heightened emotional interplay? I'll bet the answers to these questions will keep you at work decreasing undue reserve for further weeks or months, until you have eliminated it entirely.

3. Pay attention to people *emotionally*. Experts in human relations talk about "listening with the third ear." But there's more to emotional awareness than that. If you want to enjoy more intense emotional interplay with your friends and loved ones, plus the deepened relationships which shared emotions soon create, you need to build greater all-around awareness of what others feel. Not *intellectual* awareness—you don't need to give names to what you sense, or delve into psychologic causes. What counts is feeling in the gut—awareness from your own emotional or primitive, untaught acumen. This comes mainly from concern about other people as *people*, plus the habit of observing how they sit, stand and move, what tone of voice they use, tautness or relaxation about the mouth, and all the other clues which your whole life has taught you how to interpret, if only you will take the trouble to collect them.

4. Put yourself in your friend's place. In Minnesota's frozen winters, an indoor game like squash has great appeal. In squash, you stand almost side by side with racquets in hand, and alternate in hitting the ball toward the court's front wall.

When I first started to play squash, I never knew just where my opponent was aiming. By the time I could tell where the ball was going, it was often too late to reach it. So I started to mimic my opponent as he took each stroke: as the ball approached him and he started his swing, I would make exactly similar movements. I could almost always tell exactly where he was aiming before his racquet came close to the ball, and got a head start toward every shot.

Often, you get the same advantage from putting yourself in someone else's place during an emotional experience. If you observe his situation, pay close attention to his early response, and put yourself into the same posture in your mind's eye, you'll find yourself a long jump ahead. Like body movements, emotions can't be analyzed sufficiently fast to do you any good, but they can be appreciated and can call forth proper response if you go through the motions yourself for a few moments.

Build closeness—and use it. Closer friendships and loves come from shared emotion. They also give their greatest benefits through shared emotion. As you let down the barriers of reserve and build your talent for sentimental awareness, you'll find many pathways opened between you and your friends or loved ones which were not there before. But you will not enjoy the full tonic effect of a web of human relationships unless you willingly share your joys and troubles. Do things together, discuss problems together, recount experiences which the others could not actually share. You'll find the leaven of other people's concern a fine refresher when things are going well, and an unexcelled support and bracer when things are going wrong.

GOD'S LOVE

Lastly—and fittingly the final tonic and refresher in this book —there is a form of love to which you can turn by day or night, for refreshment after a weary day or for new strength in unendurable turmoil. God's love and His concern. Let that love constantly undergird you. Enjoy its refreshing power often through prayer.

Faith invigorates body, mind and soul. It is the crowning tonic, the refresher without peer.

CHAPTER FOURTEEN'S MAIN POINTS

Mind-refreshers *differ* from your ordinary activities, and *captivate* your interest. Creative diversions give extra benefits, and need not require training, expensive equipment, or special skill. *Crafts* divert some people effectively, while puzzles or problems divert others. *Pets* give sound diversion. *Tricks of mind* deserve a trial. *Partial diversions* also have a place.

Emotional outlets can help you to blow off steam and shuck off lasting turmoil. Violent physical acts against balls, targets, bowling pins and the like give considerable feeling of release. Specifically thinking about the people who caused resentment while you stab, shoot or strike gives extra aid. You can also air. your feelings through conversation. Friends and family provide confidants for mild, day-by-day difficulties. Visit specialized counselors for big issues. Prayer, later-destroyed letters, and creative outlets work out best in the middle ground.

Friendships and loves give tremendous additional strength and uplift. Potential sharing of emotion measures your involvement with another person, and offers its own rewards. You build closeness by open-heartedness and awareness—by seeking "shared-feeling" experiences, letting most emotion flow forth unrestrained, paying attention to people *emotionally,* and putting yourself in the other fellow's place. Once built, don't hesitate to "use" friendships—not for business and material ends, but for shared day-by-day living, emotional support, and frequent, intimate companionship. Finally, remember the greatest, most readily available source of love for all—God's love. Let it undergird you constantly.

Index